Suzanne Somers'
EAT GREAT,
LOSE WEIGHT

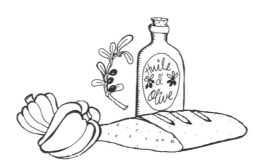

Suzanne Somers'
EAT GREAT, LOSE WEIGHT

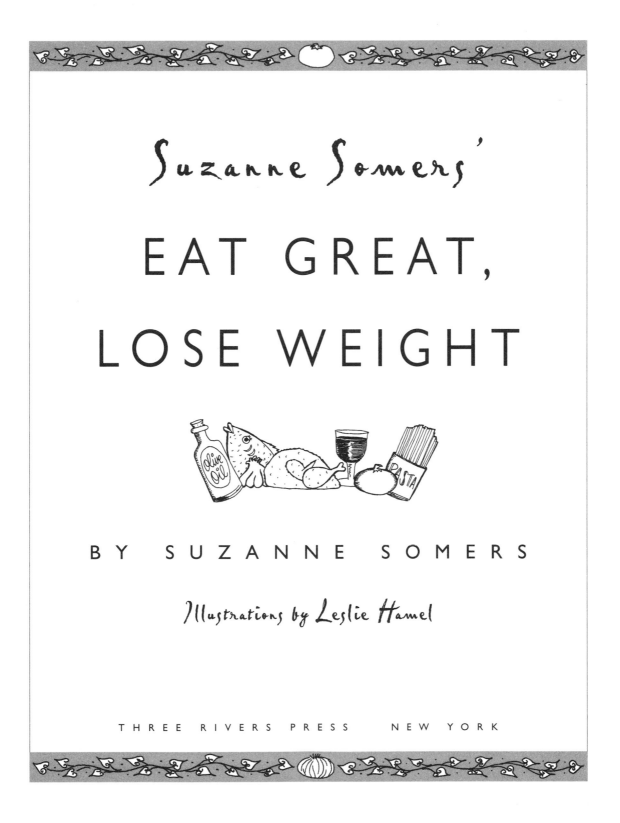

BY SUZANNE SOMERS

Illustrations by Leslie Hamel

THREE RIVERS PRESS   NEW YORK

Copyright © 1996 by Suzanne Somers

Published by Three Rivers Press, 201 East 50th Street
New York, New York 10022.
Member of the Crown Publishing Group.

Originally published in hardcover by Crown Publishers, Inc., in 1996.
First paperback edition printed in 1999.

Random House, Inc. New York, Toronto, London, Sydney, Auckland

www.randomhouse.com

THREE RIVERS PRESS and colophon are trademarks of Crown Publishers, Inc.

Printed in the United States of America

Book design by Lauren Dong and Debbie Glasserman

Library of Congress Cataloging-in-Publication Data
Somers, Suzanne
[Eat great, lose weight]
Suzanne Somers' eat great, lose weight / by Suzanne Somers.
Includes index.
1. Reducing diets   I. Title.
RM222.2.S655   1997
613.2'5—dc20   96-33178
CIP

ISBN 0-609-80058-2

10   9   8   7   6   5   4   3   2   1

First Paperback Edition

Another great idea, Al!

I love you!

And thank you, Caroline.

I love you, too!

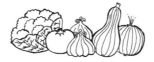

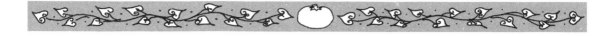

Acknowledgments

The biggest thank-you goes to Caroline Somers, my darling daughter-in-law. She spent countless hours researching for me, which made the writing of this book possible. *I* can tell you that this program works for *me,* but you also need to know why; thus, the research. Over the years, Caroline and I have connected in an incredible way through our love of food and cooking. So many of the family pictures in this book are of food preparation in the kitchen. You'll notice that, in many of them, Caroline is by my side or I am on her team, putting together some sumptuous meal for all of us. So, thank you sweet Caroline for your talent and for caring so much.

The next big thank-you goes to Alan, my wonderful husband. I was madly in love with him when I met him, and although I never thought it could be possible, I'm even crazier about him today. I love to cook for him. He is such an appreciative audience and I must give him credit for the *idea* that this would be a great book because it's the way we really eat! So, without his urging, I don't know if this book would have been written . . . I'd be too busy cooking.

Thank you, sweet Bruce, for all the favors with your computer. You have an enviable knowledge of the technical world and I know at times we take advantage of you. You are the best son! I love you and it's great being your "ma."

Then there's Leslie, my cool and fabulous stepdaughter. I gave her the assignment to "do her thing" and Somersize through art. Her wit and style come through when you look at those "angry little potatoes." She is always clever and sly in her work. We have had wonderful and loving experiences together for two decades. For many years, she has designed my costumes for Las Vegas. When I presented my act at the Sporting Club in Monte Carlo, the audience gasped in astonishment and approval at the beautiful gowns. Thanks, Les! You did it again.

And what fun it was to work with my adorable agent, Al Lowman. Thanks, Al. You are a great combination of chutzpah and vulnerability. We will be friends long after this book . . . and thanks for setting me up with the *perfect* publisher.

Every book needs a great editor, so Crown sent me their finest—the cookbook queen, Wendy Hubbert. She had the nasty assignment of coming to Saint-Tropez (where I was vacationing) and editing with me. As with all editors, there were times I wanted to strangle her, but in the end, she was right! Thank you, Wendy, for your talent and for keeping me focused when I

would rather have been dancing. You did a great job!

As always, thanks to Marsha, Wendy, and Michelle, my office "pals," for all the typing, running, and caring.

Last but probably most important, thank you to the nutritionists who put the validating stamp on this program. Without your voices I would not have the proper understanding to explain why and how this eating system works. Thank you for your time and caring: Teresa Olsen and Jay Wild, registered nutritionists; Vicky Newell, certified nutrition counselor; and Fred Garcia, M.D., Ph.D. And a very special thank-you to Barbara Dixon, L.D.N., R.D., for reviewing this book and writing the foreword. Your validation is very important to this project.

About the Photographs . . .

I'm very proud of the photographs in this book. They were taken at my beloved desert home of twenty years, a place the public has rarely seen. The recipes are very personal, creatively, so I felt it important to photograph them in the setting where they are most often served.

Everyone involved worked so hard, starting with Jeff Katz, my first choice as a photographer. Jeff is an unbelievably great talent who makes a chocolate cake look so delectable, you can taste it when you see the pictures, and then a moment later takes my picture and makes me feel like I'm the only person in the world he'd like to photograph. I'm sure everyone he shoots feels this

way, which is why he is one of the most sought-after photographers in the entertainment business. Big thank-yous to Jeff's team: Victor, Jack, and Andy.

To Donna Glennon, my creative friend who has been with me since my talk show and who has a way of dressing the set to look simple yet bountiful. And thank-you to her team: Rio and Jan.

And once again, Caroline, who cooked her brains out with me for two solid days. She is an incredible talent and perfectionist, and we had a great time in the kitchen together in spite of the heat.

All the china, silver, and crystal in the photographs belong to me, the result of twenty years of collecting. I cannot pass up a beautiful antique plate; and in my travels I am always drawn to some wondrous object (which has to be hand-carried on the airplane); but after I get it home, it becomes not only useful art but also a memory.

Linens are my other great love. My guests always talk about my sheets and linens, which gives me great pleasure. At night when all the rooms are occupied, I slip into my smooth antique sheets, smiling and content, knowing everyone in the house is experiencing the same luxury. The linens and lace panels in the color photos of me in the insert are a result of years of combing through antiques markets looking for the gorgeous (and hard-to-find) lace embroidery on tuille that is traditionally found on windows in the great houses and chateaus of Europe. Every lace panel is a work of art and represents memories of all the different and wonderful trips Alan and I have taken together.

The holiday photo (taken in 110 degrees of scorching desert heat) is especially thrilling. The dried flowers on the mantle make me smile—every bouquet originated in my garden and the flowers were once

throughout the house at all times of the year. It makes me sad to see flowers die, but I hang them upside down right before they start to fade, and because of the low humidity in the desert, they dry perfectly in a week while still retaining their color. Each bouquet is a memory and adds to a home filled with good feelings.

The antique linen napkins—sixteen of them in perfect condition—were a find. They happen to be more than a hundred years old. I love them because they are so large (24 inches square) and the fabric gets more luxurious with each passing year.

This book is an honest representation of how I really live, and the photographs give you a peek into a part of my life that I rarely share. Home, family, good food, good health, great love, and memories are what it's all about and are my reason for being. Perhaps the pictures will turn you on to the eating plan and lifestyle that have brought me inner peace and outward satisfaction. It is a pleasure to share my personal program with you. I hope you enjoy the photos and the information contained in this book as much as I've enjoyed putting them together.

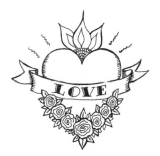

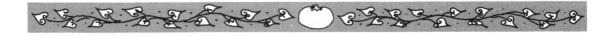

Contents

Part Two - The Somersize Recipes • 65

Ten: The Somersize Pantry • 67

Eleven: Level One: Let's Get Cookin' • 71

Dips, Spreads, and Appetizers • 73

Side Dishes (That Can Make a Meal) • 89

Salads • 105

Contents

Soups and Sandwiches • 123

Meatless Main Dishes • 137

Fish and Seafood • 147

Poultry • 155

Meat • 173

Desserts • 185

Twelve: Level Two: Keep on Cookin'! • 189

Afterword • 201

Index • 203

Foreword

By Barbara M. Dixon, L.D.N., R.D.,
nutritionist, author, and health educator

Throughout the ages, food has been a focus of our daily life. Food is satisfying, and it's associated with our memorable events: births, deaths, religious ceremonies, weddings, holidays, and personal accomplishments. Yet "over-indulgence" in food contributes to a variety of not-so-pleasurable side effects.

We Americans know this all too well; we are the most well fed people on earth. We enjoy abundance: food is everywhere and there seems to be no end to offering more and more in supermarkets and restaurants. It's no wonder we're a nation plagued with obesity and a host of digestive problems. There are likely as many remedies for obesity as for heartburn, indigestion, gas, belching, and bloating. And there's an abundance of published literature and research on these health problems. But are we alleviating our national problem of obesity and intestinal difficulties?

The answer is no. Americans are getting fatter and the availability and sales of products for indigestion continue to soar. And we continue to spend lots of money hoping that things will improve. Each year Americans spend billions of dollars on methods to counteract obesity. We also spend millions in health-food stores and in pharmacies on products such as antacids and antigas, anti-diarrheal, and anticonstipation agents to prevent or control digestive problems.

Could the solutions to these health problems lie in what we eat, when we eat, how much we eat, and how our body uses the food we eat for nourishment and energy? I think so. And you'll read more about this in the pages to come. However, there's still a lot more we need to know about the effects of food on our overall health. Fortunately, the amount of medical and nutrition research is at an all-time high.

We know that certain foods can alter our

moods, promote good health, protect us against or prevent disease, help our medications work better, and give us energy to enhance our athletic performance. Both professionals and nonprofessionals in the health field have theories regarding the role food plays in good or poor health. Some of these people have been criticized, some have sold millions of books, and some have been labeled "experts" and authorities on the subject. What we have to remember is that, like medicine, nutrition is a science that fosters differences of opinion and in research results.

Personally, I keep an open mind when it comes to the pursuit of good health. Whether answers come from our country or internationally, by professional or lay sources, I'm willing to listen, dissect the information, and come to a conclusion as to whether an approach is sound or unsound. Like most of you, I'm also interested in learning what can help us have long, abundant lives or maintain healthy bodies with plenty of energy and vitality. And, like most of you, I often look to those in the public eye—television and film celebrities, professional athletes, performers/musicians—because they are so visible that their health and physical condition can't go unnoticed. The success of their careers depends on good physical health.

Suzanne Somers is one very good example. Have you ever wondered how she does it? I must admit, I was curious myself. Aside from keeping her physical body in great shape, I wondered, What does she eat? Through this book, I became aware of her approach to healthy eating. As you'll learn,

Suzanne believes strongly in eating a variety of foods in digestive-appropriate combinations. This approach (food combining) has been practiced for many, many years and is advocated publicly by many individuals, including Professor Arnold Ehret, Herbert Shelton, Marilyn and Harvey Diamond and Dick Gregory, and Dr. John Demartini. Even orthodox Jews practice food combining in their dietary laws, by refraining from eating meat and milk dishes at the same time. And personally, my mother and aunt would remind me when I was a young child not to eat certain foods together because they would make me sick. Since I figured they had experienced the side effects of such food and beverage combinations, I avoided them as suggested.

No, food combining is not new! However, Suzanne has learned to take the basic principles of food combining and tailor them to fit her lifestyle. She's found that, for her, it is this way of *eating*—not *dieting*—that helps her maintain a healthy weight.

I have to admit, I had some concerns about this type of program used to encourage weight loss or maintenance. My initial questions were, Is the program sound or does it contribute to nutritional deficiencies? Are there individuals who should not choose this way of eating, because of existing health problems? Does the program really lead to weight loss, even with more liberal, less restrictive choices in food? And is there any scientific foundation to support the benefit of food combining for healthy digestion? Further, I wanted to know if this program encouraged exercise, gradual weight loss, behavioral modification (changing eating habits for life), and a "balanced" diet, including a variety of foods in moderate amounts.

After reviewing Ms. Somers' manuscript, all of my questions were answered. I'd like to share those answers with you.

First, as you'll learn, Somersizing (as Suzanne appropriately refers to this program) suggests you eat a variety of foods. A limited variety is certainly not an issue here; the focus is on selecting foods that can be eaten at the same time. On a daily basis, a wide choice of foods is suggested in meal plans and menus and recipes. She includes meat, chicken, seafood, vegetables, fruits, grains, dairy, and fats . . . all of which can be included in a healthy diet.

Suzanne doesn't place emphasis on exact quantities of foods you're limited to eat, but the portions and types of foods she suggests should satisfy the average nutritional requirements. (If you want to make certain you are meeting your daily nutritional needs or Recommended Daily Allowances [RDA], use the USDA-based Food Pyramid as a guide. The Food Pyramid illustrates the ranking of categories of foods by their importance in the diet.) In your daily intake, try to include at least six to eleven servings of breads, cereals, grains; two to four servings of fruits; three to five servings of vegetables; two to three servings of meat, poultry, fish, beans, and meat substitutes; two to three servings of dairy products; and limited servings of fat (choose polyunsaturated and monounsaturated fats more often than saturated fats).

I think you get the picture: a variety of "properly combined foods" can meet your nutritional needs. Therefore, you can easily adopt this way of eating without fear of nutritional deficiencies. As with any program intended for the general public, this program is not modified or restricted in foods and amounts that are appropriate for those with various health problems, including diabetes, hypoglycemia, heart disease, or coronary artery disease (with elevated total blood cholesterol, LDL cholesterol, and triglyceride levels), hypertension (high blood pressure), and renal (kidney) disease. If you have these or other health problems and have been encouraged to follow a specially prescribed diet given to you by a physician, registered dietitian, or nutritionist, please check with him or her before starting this program.

Regarding the weight-loss component of the program: Suzanne and others following this program say they have lost weight and are able to maintain their weight losses. Suzanne credits this weight loss to better digestion of foods due to eating foods that are properly combined. We nutritionists know that digestion is a complex normal body function and that each type of food is digested differently. Digestion actually begins in the mouth, where the teeth grind food and digestive juices begin breaking it down, making it easier to swallow. Then, food particles go to the stomach and are mixed with digestive "juices" (hydrochloric acid, lipase, gastrin and protease, among others) to further break down foods for more complete digestion. The stomach is normally emptied of food about one to four hours after a meal, depending on the amounts and kinds of food eaten. When eaten alone, carbohydrates leave the stomach and are ready for further digestion first and most rapidly, followed by protein, then fat. A mixed diet (containing carbohydrates, proteins, and fats) stays in the stomach longer before it empties. Food particles then enter the small and large intestines, where absorption of nutrients (vitamins and minerals, amino acids, sugars, and fats) takes place. Healthy digestion means that the body receives all the nutrients it needs and eliminates that which the body doesn't need, in the form of waste (feces), which is passed out of the body without discomfort or delay.

Does more efficient digestion mean dietary "excesses" don't matter?

Well, while I'd agree that efficient digestion is extremely important, so is setting limitations on the amounts of foods you eat. Keeping your diet simple rather than eating lots of different combinations of foods can certainly help prevent indigestion and the discomfort associated with it. Overeating creates problems, too; it makes you feel uncomfortable and can contribute to weight gain. A perfect example of abusing both the amounts and kinds of foods you eat often occurs during the holidays . . . with endless banquet tables, and a morning after you're not likely to forget. Some people eat like this on a regular basis!

When it comes to the chief contributors to being overweight or obese, energy input versus energy output ranks high. Simply put, if you take in more energy from food than you use, or "burn," for normal body functions, you will gain weight! While this program focuses on food combinations for better digestion, this doesn't mean that you should eat more foods than you need. Moderation is the key. Suzanne suggests you eat "until you are comfortable and satisfied" . . . not stuffed! Moderation is important for weight loss. Somersizing emphasizes lots of vegetables, fruits (eaten alone), and whole-grain complex carbohydrates (terrific sources of fiber). These foods are great for good elimination and fill you up, too! Avoiding foods containing large amounts of sugars is also a good idea for those seeking weight loss.

Is fat an issue in weight management? Definitely! You don't have to eliminate fat from your diet altogether, but keeping the amount of fat you eat to moderate amounts is important in helping reduce your risk of heart disease and certain forms of cancer. Watch the amount of animal products you eat because they are high in cholesterol, and getting too much raises blood cholesterol levels. If remembering percentages for fat in the diet is boring to you—as it is for Suzanne—you'll find it easy to simply avoid fried foods, to limit the amount of fat you add to foods, and to look for "hidden" fats in snack foods, whole fat dairy products, and salad dressings and sauces. The bottom line is that combining foods for good digestion is a great idea, but remember, as Suzanne does, that moderate eating and listening to your body help bring about weight loss.

What about exercise? Exercise and physical activity is important in achieving and maintaining weight loss. We know Suzanne exercises—just look at those thighs! Suzanne's approach is to make sure she gets *enjoyment* out of her physical activity. She doesn't like rigid exercise programs; neither do I, nor do most people I counsel. Whether you walk, run, swim, bike, hike, aerobic dance, or climb the stairs in your home, the idea is to keep moving every day. Physical activity enhances good digestion, relieves stress, and increases your metabolism.

The nature and causes of obesity are still puzzling to us. That's why intensive, continuing research is so important. Environment, genetics, culture, diet, and metabolism are all important contributors, and maybe one day we'll truly conquer our nation's obesity problem.

Could planning meals with combinations of foods that improve digestion, absorption, and elimination be the answer? It very well may be. In her book, Suzanne Somers is willing to share this way of eating—with lots of recipes and meal suggestions—that helps her maintain her healthy weight and gives her an abundance of energy.

Should you give it a try? Why not? Somersizing contains all the important elements of a sound weight-loss program: variety in food choices, gradual weight loss, and components for maintaining a desired weight. It encourages changes in eating habits for life, it doesn't severely restrict your calorie intake, and it encourages physical activity.

Suzanne makes the principles of food combining easy to follow and utilize when eating out in restaurants, or at social gatherings, or when preparing meals at home. If her program works for you, I hope you'll let Suzanne know. After all, *eating great* and *losing weight* is a combination we'd all like to experience!

Suzanne Somers'
EAT GREAT,
LOSE WEIGHT

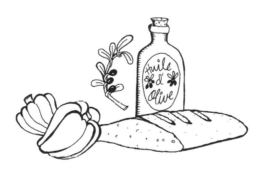

INTRODUCTION

How It All Began . . .

Many years ago, when I was just starting out in television, I landed a guest-starring role on a hit series called *Starsky and Hutch*. It was a huge break for me; I was a single mother who had just moved to Los Angeles to get my career started, and this was a week's worth of work at a time when I desperately needed the money. Three days before I was supposed to start, I got a call from the producer. My ears perked up when I heard his voice. He told me that he and the director had been sitting around talking, and they decided I was just "a little too chunky" for the part. They recast the role and I cried myself to sleep. I was twenty-nine years old and twenty pounds overweight.

That's when my diet roller coaster began. Determined to lose those pounds, I tried every diet in the world. Remember the TWA stewardess diet? You lose ten pounds in four days—unless you pass out first. Oh yes, and the waterman diet; that was a lot of laughs. You consume only meat and water for two weeks. I had horrible dog's breath and was constantly on edge . . . wonder why! Another diet I tried involved choking down this gelatinous intestinal cleanser—gag city. Or what about the four-day diet where on Day 1 you eat nine bananas; Day 2, nine oranges; Day 3, nine hot dogs; Day 4, nine bananas. Terribly convenient at a business lunch.

I tried them all! The shakes, the calorie counting, the packaged foods, the fasting, the grapefruit, the cottage cheese, the celery . . . and guess what? They all worked. That's right. Every time I went on a diet, I lost weight. *But,* within a short time of going back to eating like a normal person, I would gain back all the weight and often a little extra. Then I'd scour the fashion magazines for the next dieting trend, and off I'd go on my path toward deprivation—all in the name of being thin.

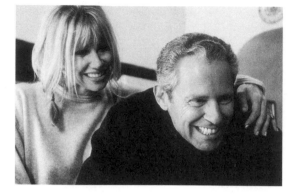

Alan and I looking happily into the future.

My diet roller coaster continued for many years. I had come to think that depriving myself of foods that I loved was a way of life. This was a huge sacrifice for me! I consider eating to be one of life's great pleasures. I have always loved to cook for myself and my family. My most treasured moments in life revolve around family gatherings, with wonderful spreads of food. Preparing food for my family and friends is the way I express my love for them. My romance with my husband, Alan, began in the kitchen, preparing incredible meals for one another. My son, Bruce, was an adventurous eater from the time he was a little boy. He would devour linguine with steamed fresh clams at the age of four. And although it took a while to win the affection of my stepchildren, Leslie and Stephen, they liked my cooking right away!

On and off the diets I went. I had no choice. Keeping control of my weight was essential to my career. The lovable Chrissy from *Three's Company* wore clothing that didn't leave much to the imagination. So I became accustomed to dieting. I suffered through the bland foods, the dismal portions, and the constant hunger. After a period of deprivation, I would reward myself with rich foods like cake and chocolate and all the others things I loved. I have always had a hearty appetite. Bruce used to call me Mr. Ed, after the horse, because I could outeat him and all of his friends.

But it seemed that right about the time I hit forty, things began to change. My metabolism slowed down and it became harder than ever to control my weight. The diets were no longer effective. Suddenly I grew hips with handles and my thighs would rub together when I walked. After I would eat a meal my stomach would bloat, and there seemed to be no way to hold it in. I found myself buying control-top panty hose to hold in that tummy. I continued the dieting and the deprivation, but I was getting fewer and fewer results. I remember Joan Rivers making a joke that I would be a good candidate for liposuction. Ouch!

The year 1992 was when everything changed. My revelation began on a trip to France for my stepson's wedding. Alan's son, Stephen, had met a wonderful French woman named Olivia, and they were to be married in her hometown—a small, medieval stone village in central France.

Our whole family made the trip from Los Angeles. Alan and I went early and were later joined by Bruce and his wife, Caroline, my stepdaughter, Leslie, and her best friend, Brigid.

The first night at Olivia's was magical. She and her family were positively charming—consummate hosts, and very bright and interesting people. They made us feel extremely welcome at their spectacular home, which was on the hillside of a valley. Each room was a stone bungalow connected to the outdoors by a stone staircase and pathway. The garden was in full May bloom. The table was set outside on the patio, under a cherry tree dripping with beautiful ripe cherries.

Olivia's mother, Mizou, prepared an outstanding meal. We started with a superb pâté served on a bed of greens dressed lightly with lemon, garlic, and extra-virgin olive oil. The entrée was a beautiful piece of lotte (a French white fish) in a butter and wine sauce, accompanied by an assortment of fresh spring vegetables. Every bite was to die for. (To this day I consider Mizou one of the best cooks I know. She makes simple foods, using the best ingredients available, and she prepares them to perfection.) After dinner the cheese tray was passed: from the ripest triple creams, like Saint Felician, to an aged Stilton, to a firm Port-Salut. A basket of breads accompanied the cheese: whole-grain toast points and chewy French sourdough. And, of course, dessert was yet to come. It was a dark-chocolate mousse served with whipped cream. Simple. Elegant. Unbelievably delicious.

Each course was complemented by selections from Olivia's father's extensive collection of wines. Her father, Jean Pierre Fougeirol, buys and sells chateaus in Mirmande, France. One of the benefits of his business is that, when he buys a chateau, he is often given the wine before selling the property to the next owner. His selections for our first dinner together were incredible. The wine tasted divine, like drinking nectar from the gods. It perfectly accentuated the flavor of the food.

We chatted long into the evening, conversing in both French and English. I struggled with my broken French; however, it improved dramatically with each sip of wine! Fortunately, Olivia's family speaks almost perfect English.

After a thoroughly enchanting evening, we gathered our coats and began saying good-bye to our new extended family. We stood under the cherry tree and I plucked a cherry from one of the branches and popped it into my mouth. It burst with flavor. The cherries were so unbelievably good that soon all of us were stuffing our faces. After devouring all the cherries within reach, Bruce hopped onto Alan's back to reach a little higher into the tree. Stephen brought a chair and Leslie stood on it to gather a few more handfuls.

Suddenly Jean Pierre appeared from the house and bellowed a warning in his thick French accent: "You must not eat zee cherries!" We were like kids caught with their hands in the cookie jar! I had to spit out the three or four pits in my mouth before I could ask why. My God, were they covered in pesticides? "No," he explained. "Do not eat the cherries! If you eat the cherries after your dinner, you will experience horrible indigestion. You will get zee gas something awful."

And was he ever right! All night long we tossed and turned. My stomach was distended and I felt extremely uncomfortable. I thought about the cherry warning, but I assumed I was feeling bad because of the cheese and the wine and the butter sauce and all of the rich food we'd eaten. I remember thinking, How can the French eat such rich food and stay so thin? I could never survive for any length of time in France. I would be as big as a house if I lived there.

The next day I asked Jean Pierre about his warning, and he explained the basic premises of food combining to me. Fruit can upset the digestive process when eaten with other foods. Therefore, he told me, I should always eat fruit on an empty stomach. He went on to explain that protein or fats should not be combined with carbohydrates. I thought about the meal we had eaten the night before and realized there were very few carbohydrates. Bread was passed with the pâté course and the cheese course, but Olivia's parents did not take any; they ate their cheese with a knife and fork.

Jean Pierre then explained that protein and fats are easily digested when eaten with vegetables only, and that carbohydrates should be eaten in their whole-grain form without any fats at all. This method of food combining is common in France, where people routinely combine their foods to keep their digestive tracts working smoothly and their weight under control without sacrificing flavor. "You mean to tell me that I can eat pâté and salad

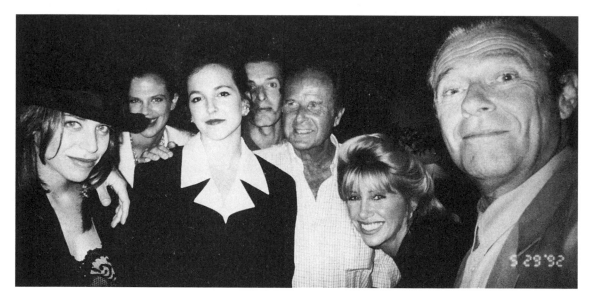

The night we all met Jean Pierre Fougeirol—Leslie, Caroline, Jean Pierre, me, and Alan.

and fish with lemon butter sauce and vegetables and cheese and wine and chocolate and still lose weight?" It sounded too good to be true! This was something that required further investigation.

When I returned home to the States, I started my quest to learn about food combining. The basic concept has been around for many years. It was developed in the 1800s and was later denounced in the mid-1900s. It came back to the forefront of the weight-loss movement in the 1970s, with *Fit for Life* and *Dr. Atkins' Diet Revolution*. I tried *Fit for Life,* and although I agreed with the basic principles and I did lose weight, I couldn't stay on it for any length of time. It was much too restrictive. I ate mostly fruit and vegetables, very little protein, and almost no fat. Deprivation, deprivation, deprivation! Dr. Atkins' plan was full of flavor, but too restrictive in carbohydrates. There was so much protein and fat on the program that even though I lost weight, I felt terribly unhealthy eating such high quantities of meat and fat—even though they were combined correctly. My objective was to find a way to eat healthy, nutritious, yet flavorful foods in substantial portions and still lose weight.

I'm happy to tell you I have found it. After working with many nutritionists, reading several books, and practicing trial and error on my own body, I have finally found a way to control my weight without deprivation. I call my program "Somersizing," and Somersizing is *not* a diet. *Diet* is a nasty four-letter word that conjures up negative thoughts of sacrifice and obsession and guilt. Somersizing is a lifestyle that will change your way of thinking about how to lose weight and how to increase your energy. Eating the Somersize way is a pleasure. It is a program for life, a program I will happily live on for the rest of *my* life. There are a few basic rules you will learn, and then you're free to eat whatever you want, in a restaurant, at home, or on the road.

Food is only one component of a happy, healthy life. I firmly believe that you must master not only your physical health but also your emotional wellness. In this book, I'll show you what works for me. You'll learn how to be fit, not fanatic; how to make movement and fitness a pleasurable part of daily life; how to make the most of every moment of every day, including your meals.

Since I started properly combining my foods, I have trimmed down from 130 to 116 pounds—the amount I weighed as a teenager. And since I reached my goal weight, I have fluctuated no more than 3 pounds. I eat delicious foods—I eat cheese, I drink wine occasionally, and you would be shocked to know how much chocolate I eat and still maintain my weight. My husband, Alan, started Somersizing, and he lost fifteen pounds and significantly lowered his cholesterol. My daughter-in-law, Caroline, gave birth to my beautiful granddaughter last October. Caroline gained forty pounds during the pregnancy. Within seven weeks she had Somersized her way back down to a size four. And Alan's daughter, Leslie, lost those last ten "hard to lose" pounds on this program. Recently Leslie married a wonderful Frenchman named Frank Buffa, a personal trainer and former Mr. France.

Frank has used food combining for years, and he and Leslie have helped numerous clients lose weight with Somersizing. My sister Maureen has been resisting me for several years. Finally I convinced her to try Somersizing, and she lost ten pounds in the first two weeks! My eighty-one-year-old mother is Somersizing to help her digest food more easily. And as for those of my initially doubtful friends who tried Somersizing with hesitation, they too were knocked out by the results: they've lost ten, fifteen, twenty pounds, and more.

How can it be so easy? How can I possibly be losing weight when I am eating more than ever before? My accountant has dieted all his life. He lost twenty pounds in one month and calls Somersizing the easiest way to lose weight he's ever tried. My neighbor Irv lost twenty-seven pounds on the program. He hates to diet and he hates to count calories. Somersizing is perfect for him. In fact, everyone with whom I have shared this program has had dramatic results for the better, and they have all urged me to share Somersizing with you.

Many experts will argue that food combining is a myth—a calorie is a calorie and it doesn't matter how you combine them, it only matters how many you eat and how many you burn off. The debate has gone on for many years, and I'm sure it will continue for many more. Say what you want about food combining. All I can tell you is that it works for me. I can eat all the wonderful foods I love and still lose weight. I don't have to give up flavor. I don't settle for boring meals with no sauce. I enjoy rich and flavorful foods. I don't count calories or fat grams. "Calorie, Smalorie," that's what I say. And after you try Somersizing and see and feel the results of this simple and satisfying way of life, I'm sure you will agree.

Throw everything you think you know about diets out the window. Somersizing is an easy and effective way to look and feel your best while enjoying life to the fullest. You'll have more energy than ever before; you'll say good-bye to the bloating and gas that used to routinely follow mealtimes; and you'll lose weight.

I put this book together to show you how I eat and to share how I cook for my family. I've compiled more than a hundred of my favorite Somersize recipes for you to try for yourself—everything from Thanksgiving Turkey with Mushroom Sausage Stuffing to Decadent Chocolate Cake—and I'm sure you will agree that this is a sinfully delightful way to *Eat Great, Lose Weight*. Enjoy!

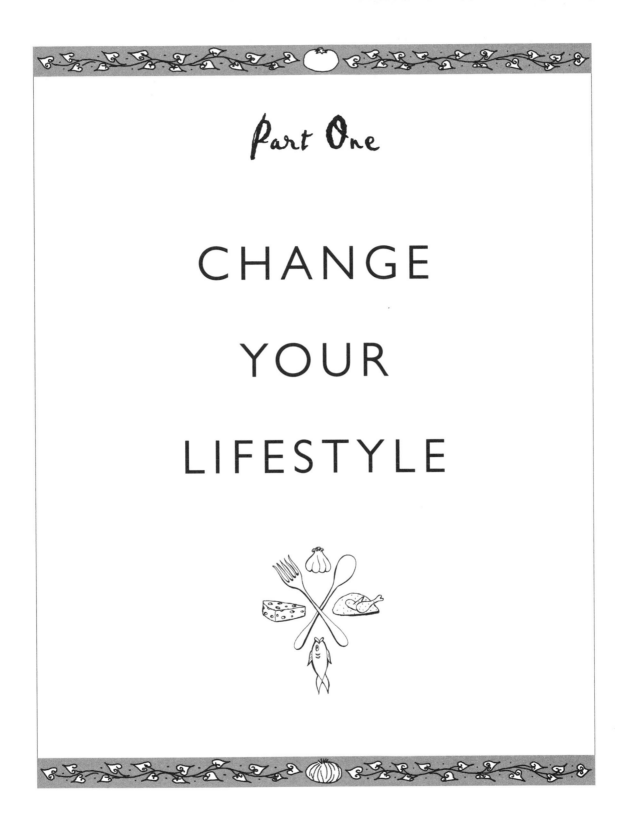

Part One

CHANGE

YOUR

LIFESTYLE

CHAPTER ONE

Diets Don't Work

You've heard it a thousand times. Most diets fail because they are based on deprivation. After depriving yourself for a period of time, you will eventually want to reward yourself. During the reward time, you will probably gain back the weight, and then some. The statistics are depressing: 95 percent of those who go on diets gain back all the weight they lost.

We're obviously doing something wrong.

It has to do with your metabolism: the rate at which your body burns calories for fuel. Some lucky people have a naturally high metabolism and can eat whatever they want and can still stay thin, while others with a low metabolism eat like birds and continue to have weight problems. Is it possible to change your metabolism? Of course. Yo-yo dieting can change it—for the worse. Going on and off diets can actually dangerously disrupt your system and lower your metabolism. Diets that restrict

your calorie intake *will* help you lose weight, but only temporarily. The human body is a complicated and remarkably adaptable machine.

When you start eating fewer calories, your body will initially burn off your fat reserves to make up for the missing fuel source. But as your fat stores are being depleted by dieting, your metabolism actually *slows down* to keep you from starving to death. It's the survival mechanism. Your body adapts to survive on fewer calories than it needed before.

It is at this point that your weight usually plateaus. Even though you're still faithfully sticking to your diet, you've stopped losing weight. That's when frustration sets in, and most people go back to eating the way they used to.

Here's the worst part. You now have a lower metabolism than before you started the diet, so your body needs fewer calories to survive. When you go back to eating the way you used to, not only will you gain back *all* the weight but you'll probably gain a little extra on top of it because of your newly lowered metabolism. Appetite suppressants create the same scenario: diet pills kill our appetite, so we eat less food. Eating fewer calories jump-starts the weight-loss process, but our bodies adjust to eating a smaller amount of food by lowering the metabolism to keep us from starving to death. Once again, the body's natural survival instinct swings into high gear. As soon as you go off the diet pills, your appetite returns . . . and so will all the pounds you lost.

Don't despair. Somersizing can actually *increase* your metabolism, so you can eat more food and still lose weight. My friend Maria Hoksbergen has spent most of her life starving herself in order to lose weight. She would eat only a couple of crackers for breakfast, a salad with no dressing for lunch, and a very small, bland dinner. She exercised three or four times a week; she took dance classes; and yet she could not lose those last ten stubborn pounds. Her doctors said she *should* be losing weight because her calorie intake was small, and she was burning off plenty of calories from her activities. They assumed she must be cheating and binge-eating in the closet. How could she eat so little and still not lose weight?

The problem was her metabolism. She had starved herself for so long that her system had actually adjusted to eating fewer calories. Her body never knew when it was going to get any food, so it got used to operating on many fewer calories. It held on to each nibble as future fuel, storing it as

I'm using the words diet *and* weight loss *a lot. But what Somersizing can really do —at the heart of it all—is help you learn to love food again. Food is one of the greatest pleasures in life. It is not your enemy! Yet most people approach the meal table with tension. I look forward to each and every meal. I know I'm going to eat wonderful food and enjoy the company of my friends and loved ones. I want you to be able to have this same healthy and happy outlook toward food.*

fat rather than burning it to provide her with immediate energy. When I suggested she try Somersizing, she said, "If I ate like you, I'd be as big as a cow."

After I explained how food combining works, she decided to give it a try. She started eating three times as much as she used to, but in the proper combinations. In a couple of weeks, she had lost the ten pounds, and even a few more. She had more energy to get through the day, and she could not believe she was able to eat so much rich and delicious food and still lose weight. She had reprogrammed her metabolism—another Somersizing success story!

Chances are, if you're reading this book, you, too, have had less than successful results

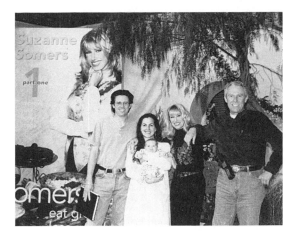

My son Bruce, daughter-in-law Caroline, granddaughter Camelia, me, and Alan on the set of Somersize.

with diets. With Somersizing, you never have to diet again. This is a new approach to eating—no starvation, no bloating or cramping after meals, and increased energy.

THE SKINNY ON FAT

In the last decade, fat has been portrayed as the major villain leading to poor health and excess weight. We've all been watching our fat intake so we can lose that weight, right?

Well, this may come as a shock. In the last

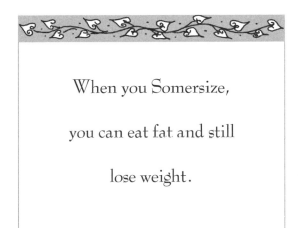

When you Somersize,

you can eat fat and still

lose weight.

decade, we Americans have cut our intake of fat from 38 to 34 percent of our daily calories, and yet we've each put on an average of eight pounds. How can that be? Isn't a reduced-fat diet supposed to help us lose weight? Doesn't less fat in our diets mean less fat on our bodies?

Not necessarily. There are other factors involved, such as whether or not you're exercising, and your energy intake versus energy expenditure. Scientists tell us that heredity and environment play important roles.

One of the first things people challenge me on when they hear about Somersizing is the fat issue. When you Somersize, you can eat cheese. You can eat a juicy steak with a mushroom cream sauce. You can eat chicken with lemon butter sauce. You can eat a taco salad topped with salsa and sour cream. You can eat tuna salad or egg salad with mayonnaise.

We've been trained to think that a diet low in fat combined with increased exercise is the *only* way to lose weight. And it's often effective. But I'm telling you that a low-fat diet does not guarantee you will lose weight. *What you are eating in place of that fat will have a lot to do with determining how much weight you lose.* Fat-free pastries, fat-free cookies, fat-free cakes, low-fat potato chips, reduced-fat crackers, fat-free caramel rice cakes, fat-free licorice, nonfat frozen yogurt—less fat? Yes. But are they your ticket to weight loss? Maybe not.

Junk food is junk food, whether it's fat free or not. It's nearly impossible to lose weight if you're filling up on these so-called *healthy* snack alternatives. Most of these products are empty foods that leave your body nutritionally unsatisfied and hungry for a decent meal. And the culprit in all of these fat-free products is . . . *sugar!* Too much sugar makes us fat. Besides the sugar, these products often have white flour and a host of chemicals that your body does not need or appreciate. I have a friend who used to eat a large nonfat frozen yogurt every day. She figured it was basically a "free food," since it was low in calories and had no fat. She couldn't figure out why she was gaining weight. I explained that it was the sugar. In my opinion, sugar is the body's greatest enemy—and is an even worse cul-

prit than fat when it comes to weight loss. You'll learn all about it in the next few chapters.

Believe it or not, you can have fat in your diet in moderation. I think that's the main reason Somersizing has been so successful with everyone who has tried it. You can incorporate rich, flavorful foods into your healthy diet and still lose the weight you want—and that helps people stick to the program.

Please don't misunderstand what I'm saying. I'm not suggesting you go out and gorge on fat. Quite the contrary. I watch my fat intake carefully because a diet low in fat has many health benefits, including a decreased risk of heart disease and some types of cancer. I choose lean meats. I cook in olive oil. I watch my cheese intake. Every now and then, however, I treat myself to a cheese soufflé, a butter sauce, or a piece of brie—without guilt. How wonderful not to feel deprived when you're trying to lose weight.

So if you're tired of the diet roller coaster, Somersizing will get you off that ride forever. It works for me. It can work for you, too.

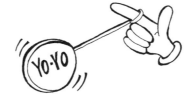

CHAPTER TWO

Stop Dieting, Start Somersizing!

Somersizing is not a diet! I can't say that enough. Somersizing is a weight-loss solution to the diet roller coaster: it's a *lifestyle,* a whole new way of eating that will change your thinking about losing weight and gaining energy. In this chapter, I'll give you an overview of the program. We'll get into the details later.

The plan is simple. I call the weight-loss portion Level One, and the maintenance portion Level Two.

LEVEL ONE

Level One is for people who want to lose weight. It's the entry level to Somersizing, where you will learn the easy guidelines for combining foods. Here's what I might eat in a typical Level One day: a delicious Fruit Smoothie (page 88) in the morning, followed by whole wheat toast or cereal; pasta primavera or a Grilled Chicken Caesar Salad (page 117) for lunch; maybe a piece of Cheddar cheese in the afternoon as a snack; and for dinner a New York strip steak with a lovely mushroom sauce, plenty of fresh grilled vegetables, and a green salad with a creamy Roquefort dressing (page 108).

On Level One, expect to feel full, satisfied, and energized, not deprived. Expect to lose those unwanted pounds as your body adjusts to the program. Some people will lose five to ten pounds in the first couple of weeks. Others, like myself, will take longer to see the results. Be patient. Every body is different. Even if you're not concerned about weight loss, Somersizing will alleviate common digestive problems and gastric distress. Have you ever eaten a huge meal of meat and potatoes and felt bloated and uncomfortable? No longer. I travel on planes a lot, and within minutes of eating those heavy airline meals, most people

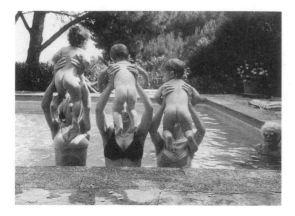

Three future Somersizers—my three grandchildren on vacation in Saint-Tropez. My mother is in the corner of the pool.

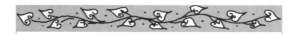

Somersizing is finding an easy,

livable way to look and feel your

best, enjoy life, eat great food,

have a healthy body you're happy

with, and have a finely tuned

digestive system and

metabolism.

around me either go to sleep, head straight for the bathroom, or begin passing gas. These are the times I wish the whole world would Somersize!

There are three important steps on Level One: (1) eliminate, (2) separate, and (3) combine. You'll learn more about these in detail, but here are the basics.

First, I *eliminate* a small list of foods that wreak havoc on our systems. These foods are called Funky Foods.

Funky Foods include sugars, high-starch foods like white flour and potatoes, caffeine, and alcohol.

Then I separate normal, everyday foods into four Somersize Food Groups: proteins and fats, vegetables, carbohydrates, and fruits. You will find complete lists of these food groups in Chapters 4 and 5.

Proteins/Fats include meat, poultry, fish, eggs, oil, butter, and cheese.

Veggies include a whole host of fresh vegetables, from artichokes to peppers to zucchini.

Carbos include whole-grain pastas, cereals, breads, beans, and nonfat dairy products.

Fruits include a huge variety of fresh fruits, from apples to peaches to tangerines.

Finally, I create exciting meals by combining these foods in Somersize combinations that aid in weight control and digestion. *I eat whenever I am hungry. I do not skimp on portions. I eat until I am full and I never skip meals.*

Here are the seven easy Somersize steps.

1. Eliminate all Funky Foods.
2. Eat Fruits alone, on an empty stomach.

3. Eat Proteins/Fats with Veggies.
4. Eat Carbos with Veggies and no fat.
5. Keep Proteins/Fats separate from Carbos.
6. Wait three hours between meals if switching from a Proteins/Fats meal to a Carbos meal, or vice versa.
7. Do not skip meals. Eat three meals a day, and eat until you feel satisfied and comfortably full.

What this means is that you can eat a Carbos and Veggies meal of whole-grain pasta and vegetables, with a whole wheat roll. But you can't add oil, chicken, or cheese because these are in the Proteins/Fats group. You can eat a Proteins/Fats and Veggies meal of fish with a butter sauce and vegetables. But you can't have any carbos like bread, rice, or pasta. Get it?

Seven steps. That's it. As long as you follow the Level One guidelines, you can eat until you are satisfied—and still lose weight.

You don't believe me, right? You probably think that, later in this book, I will reveal that you have to mix powders or take pills or count calories and fat grams, or buy special Somersize packaged foods, or fast for the first week. Not with Somersizing. Just eliminate the Funky Foods, then eat in proper combinations. That's the program. For those of you who say, "But I love Funky Foods like potatoes and sourdough rolls. And I have a real sweet tooth! I can't give those things up!" I will tell you there is no way to lose weight magically. But the benefits of the Somersize system far outweigh the restrictions. So I don't eat sugar and white bread. Look at what I *do* eat! Whole grains, fresh vegetables, fruit, a huge variety

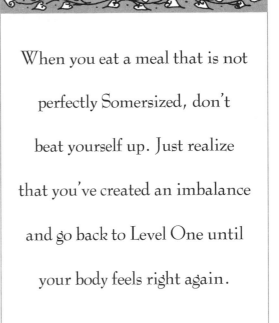

When you eat a meal that is not perfectly Somersized, don't beat yourself up. Just realize that you've created an imbalance and go back to Level One until your body feels right again.

of meats, cheese, and delicious sauces. That's right. When I want butter or cream or eggs or cheese, I eat it. Hardly a sacrifice to lose all the weight you want *and* gain vital energy.

A Sample Week

Still skeptical? I don't think about every meal with great detail—this way of eating has become second nature to me, as it will to you. To give you an example of all the combinations of food on the Somersize system, I have written down absolutely everything I ate for an entire week so you could see what constitutes a whole week's worth of meals on Level One. You'll find many of these recipes in Chapter 11.

I haven't included portion size because,

as you know, you eat until you are satisfied and comfortably full. Your meals can vary from mine tremendously, but you'll get the idea.

SUNDAY

9:00 Breakfast—Proteins/Fats and Veggies
Cheese omelet with fresh vegetables of your choice
Decaf coffee

1:00 Lunch—Carbos and Veggies
Whole-grain pasta with Simple Tomato, Basil, and Garlic Sauce (page 145) (no oil or cheese)
Cucumber Tomato Salad (page 112) dressed with lemon, salt, and pepper
Iced herbal tea

4:00 Snack—Fruits
A couple of tangerines
Water with a squeeze of lime

7:00 Family Dinner—Proteins/Fats and Veggies
Roast Chicken with Mushroom Sausage Stuffing and Tarragon Gravy (page 157)
Steamed asparagus
Butter lettuce salad with Garlic Vinaigrette (page 95)
Decaf Coffee Granita (page 187)

MONDAY

7:00 Breakfast—Fruits
Fruit Smoothie of peaches, raspberries, and orange juice (page 88)

7:20—Carbos
Whole wheat toast with nonfat cottage cheese
Decaf coffee

10:00 Snack—Fruits
Apple

1:00 Lunch—Proteins/Fats and Veggies
Grilled shrimp in butter, parsley, and lemon sauce
Grilled Chicken Caesar Salad (page 117)

4:00 Snack—Carbos
Fat-free whole wheat pretzels

7:30 Dinner—Proteins/Fats and Veggies
Chicken vegetable soup from leftovers (no rice, potatoes, pasta, or carrots)
Tricoloré Salad with Balsamic Vinaigrette (page 106)

TUESDAY

7:00 Breakfast—Fruits
Sliced mangoes and strawberries, a glass of pineapple juice

7:20—Carbos
Grape-Nuts cereal with nonfat milk

1:00 Lunch—Proteins/Fats and Veggies
Iceberg Lettuce with Roquefort Dressing (page 108)
Grilled chicken breast with assorted grilled vegetables (zucchini, onions, peppers)

7:00 Dinner—Carbos and Veggies
Brown rice with steamed vegetables (broccoli, yellow squash, red peppers), soy sauce, hot red pepper flakes
Butter lettuce salad with Fat-Free Yogurt Dressing (page 78)

9:00—Dessert
Lemon fruit sorbet (fruit juice sweetened, no added sugar), fruits

WEDNESDAY

6:00 Breakfast—Fruits
Honeydew melon

6:45—*Carbos*
    Decaf cappuccino with nonfat milk
9:00—*Carbos*
    Toasted pumpernickel bagel
    Nonfat yogurt
2:00 Lunch—*Proteins/Fats and Veggies*
    Grilled Chicken Salad with Sun-Dried
        Tomatoes and Goat Cheese
        (page 115)
6:00 Dinner—*Proteins/Fats and Veggies*
    Chicken Piccata with lemon and
        capers (page 156)
    Assorted grilled vegetables
    Radicchio, arugula, and endive salad
        with Parmesan cheese
9:00 Snack—*Proteins/Fats*
    Piece of Cheddar cheese

THURSDAY

7:00 Breakfast—*Proteins/Fats*
    Scrambled eggs with lean turkey
        sausage links
    Decaf coffee
1:00 Lunch—*Proteins/Fats and Veggies*
    Taco salad (romaine, shredded beef,
        Cheddar cheese, salsa, sour cream;
        no tortillas, beans, or guacamole)
4:00 Snack—*Carbos*
    Fat-free whole wheat pretzels
7:30 Dinner—*Proteins/Fats and Veggies*
    Broiled Sea Bass with "Candied"
        Tomatoes and Seared Escarole
        (page 151)
    Steamed Artichoke with Lemon Dill
        Mayonnaise (page 85)
9:30 Dessert—*Fruits*
    Raspberry sorbet (fruit juice
        sweetened, no sugar)

FRIDAY

9:00 Breakfast—*Fruits*
    Papaya
9:30—*Carbos*
    Shredded wheat cereal with nonfat milk
12:30 Lunch—*Proteins/Fats and Veggies*
    Cobb salad (lettuce, blue cheese, turkey,
        bacon, tomato, green onion, hard-
        boiled egg, Italian dressing; no
        avocado)
6:00 Dinner—*Proteins/Fats and Veggies*
    Green salad with Blue Cheese
        Vinaigrette (page 116)
    Ratatouille (page 101) with grilled
        chicken
    Sugarless Cheesecake (page 186)

SATURDAY

9:00 Breakfast—*Fruits*
    Fruit Smoothie (page 88)
9:20—*Carbos*
    Grape-Nuts cereal with nonfat milk
    Decaf cappuccino with nonfat milk
1:00 Lunch—*Carbos and Veggies*
    Pita Sandwich with Veggies and Yogurt
        Cheese (page 135)
    Hummus with Pita Triangles and
        Crudités (page 77)
6:30 Dinner—*Proteins/Fats and Veggies*
    Grilled Lamb Chops with Fresh Herbs
        (page 177)
    Grilled Zucchini and Eggplant
        (page 90)
    "Candied" Tomatoes (page 76)
    Green Salad with Artichoke Hearts and
        Red Wine Vinaigrette (page 107)
8:30 Dessert—*Fruits*
    Tangerines

I bet you've never eaten food like this on any "diet"! In the following chapters you'll learn more about the seven easy Somersize steps so you can enjoy delicious, flavorful foods without going hungry. You can dine in any kind of restaurant. You can cook for yourself using any of my Somersize recipes or create Somersize favorites of your own. Simple. Effective. Incredible!

LEVEL TWO

When you reach your goal weight, you will graduate to Level Two, the maintenance portion of this program. You can loosen the reins a bit and learn how to Somersize for the rest of your life—enjoying your life without worrying about your weight fluctuating more than a couple of pounds. On Level Two, you will follow the basic Level One Somersize guidelines but incorporate some Funky Foods in moderation, even including wine and chocolate in your meals.

What works for me is to eat Level One foods as a general rule. When I splurge, I realize I am creating an imbalance. I almost never eat white-flour products, even in Level Two. It just doesn't feel good in my system. Remember making glue in kindergarten? It was a mixture of white flour and water. I visualize this glue every time I eat anything made with white flour. No wonder people experience indigestion, with thick gooey glue clogging up their systems. I have learned to love whole wheat breads and pastas.

The foods in Level One are so delicious that I find it easy and livable to eat them.

There was an initial adjustment in my eating because I was raised on meat and potatoes. It was difficult at first because I was used to a "stuffed" feeling after meals. I wasn't satisfied until my stomach was sticking out and bloated. This was how I "knew" I was satisfied. When I first started Somersizing, I had to eat huge portions of food to feel full, but in time, my body adjusted to this new eating and I began to feel light and satisfied with less food.

Today, when I splurge and have some combination of protein and carbohydrates, I usually find it isn't worth it. The bloat comes back, my energy dips, I toss and turn in my sleep because of the indigestion, and elimination becomes difficult. If I do this too many days in a row, I notice weight coming back. For what? So I can have a potato with my steak?

After you have lost all the weight you desire, you can start incorporating some precisely forbidden foods into your meals. But think it through; *listen to your body.* Everybody is different. For me, I have found that most often I can have oil with my pastas and butter with my toast and it does not seem to affect my digestive system and I don't seem to gain weight. I have desserts and wine on occasion but I find that too many meals including these foods start showing up on my waistline.

If I create too many imbalances, the old symptoms reappear—bloating, gas, indigestion, yawning in the afternoon, a general dip in my energy, and weight gain. This is what I mean when I say Level Two can create imbalances. Only you will know what your body can handle. My weight now fluctuates by about three pounds. Any more than this, an alarm goes off in my head. I realize it's time to go back to Level One.

Indulgences are not for every day. The beauty of Level Two is to allow the "fun" foods we all enjoy to be a part of our lifestyle, *but* you have to understand the imbalances they create and not *overindulge* and blow all the work you've done to look and feel so good.

Level Two is an extension of Level One, with occasional treats. Moderation is the key to maintaining your weight. Some people have to stay very close to Level One guidelines, with a minor imbalance here and there, in order to maintain their weight. Others find they can create quite a few imbalances with no problem. By using trial and error on your own body, you will find out how many imbalances you can handle. You'll learn all about Level Two in Chapter 9, but here are some examples of how you can loosen the reins and still maintain your weight.

Minor Imbalances

A minor imbalance with an otherwise Level One meal would not cause much of a disruption. Most Somersizers can frequently enjoy minor imbalances on Level Two without gaining weight.

- A little fat with Carbos and Veggies meals, i.e., whole-grain pasta with vegetables sautéed in a little olive oil, with a sprinkle of Parmesan; a vegetarian sandwich with a little mayo or avocado
- A glass of wine with your meal
- A touch of sugar or flour included in your sauce or salad dressing
- Berries on whole-grain cereal or yogurt; whole-grain toast with fruit juice–sweetened berry jam on toast
- A couple squares of dark chocolate (made from at least 60 percent cocoa) between meals

Moderate Imbalances

A moderate imbalance with an otherwise Level One meal can be enjoyed every now and then. You will need to adjust for it by eating Level One meals until you get your balance back. (For some people, that may mean one meal; for others, it may mean five.)

- Whole grains combined with proteins: chicken with brown rice, fish with whole grain pasta, steak with wild rice, tuna salad on wheat bread
- Somersize (low-sugar, low-flour) desserts, i.e., flourless chocolate cake, cheesecake, tart with whole wheat crust, chocolate mousse, berries with whipped cream

Major Imbalances

These are the kinds of foods I try to stay away from completely. Make sure your indulgence is really worth it. A major imbalance, like this, should be very infrequent. After indulging, go back on Level One until you have your balance back.

- Proteins/Fats with Carbos and Funky Foods, i.e., a meatball sandwich on a white roll, a hamburger with french fries, cheese and sausage pizza with beer, sweet-and-sour pork with white rice, chicken nachos and a margarita, turkey with mashed potatoes, a candy bar, banana bread, pecan pie

Experiment to see how many imbalances you can handle. Remember to consider your portion size whenever you stray from Level One Guidelines. If you notice you are gaining a few pounds, or you feel tired and sluggish, go back to Level One until you fix the problem.

Desserts

Every now and then it's okay to enjoy a dessert in Level Two. Just stay away from desserts made with a lot of sugar or white

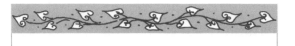

You can be in control of your weight for the rest of your life.

flour. After a Proteins/Fats meal, I might have a piece of cheesecake with fresh berries. (Cheesecake is made mostly of proteins/fats—eggs, cream cheese, sour cream, lemon juice, sugar, and sometimes a touch of flour or cornstarch.) Pudding, crème brûlée, chocolate mousse, and even ice cream are generally lower in sugar than most other desserts and, unlike most pastries, do not have white flour. Flourless chocolate cake or strawberries dipped in chocolate are also great dessert choices.

Now you have a basic overview of how to lose weight on Level One and how to maintain your weight on Level Two. But you probably still have many unanswered questions. Read the following chapters to get a full understanding of how and why Somersizing works. Trust me; you will want this information because your friends will not believe you when you tell them how you lost all those unwanted pounds while eating such great food!

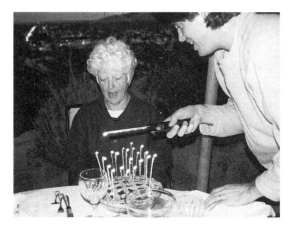

Bruce lighting the candles on my mother's eighty-first birthday pie—a whole wheat–crust berry pie.

CHAPTER THREE

Why Somersizing Works

Every person with whom I have shared this plan has had dramatic results for the better. But even after losing twenty pounds, some of them still can't understand why they are losing weight when they're eating more—and better—than ever before.

The actual physiological processes of the human body are extremely complicated. I am not a doctor or a nutritionist, but I will try to explain how Somersizing works in the layman's terms that I have come to understand from experts in diet and nutrition. Here's how Somersizing helps you lose weight and increase your energy.

YOUR BODY AND SUGAR: IT AIN'T SO SWEET

It pains me to say it, because I have a tremendous sweet tooth, but sugar is my body's greatest enemy. Surprisingly, for me

sugar can cause as much or more weight gain than fat. Of the sugar you eat, what your body doesn't use for fuel, it will save for the future as fat.

And we Americans love sugar! I was shocked when I heard that sugar makes up nearly 25 percent of the calories in the average American diet. (Some studies show that figure as high as 50 percent!) And the most unlikely carbohydrate foods are broken down into sugars in the body—carrots, beets, corn, and white bread, among other suspects.

Remember the Funky Foods? One of the most important aspects of Somersizing is the elimination of sugars and foods high in starch (such as white flour, white rice, potatoes) that turn right to sugar upon digestion.

Sugars and starches are both carbohydrates, the body's main source of fuel. Carbohydrates are easy for your body to break down, and therefore are a good source of quick energy. But some carbohydrates can cause weight problems. To understand why, let's look at what happens when you eat carbohydrates.

When you eat carbohydrates, your body breaks them down into glucose (sugar). Some of the glucose is transported via your blood cells to be burned for immediate energy. Excess glucose is transported via your blood cells to your fat cells.

So eating simple sugars and certain carbohydrates causes a rise in the level of glucose in your blood: your blood sugar level. In response to the higher amount of glucose in your blood, your pancreas secretes a hormone called insulin in order to restore your blood sugar level. Insulin carries the glucose to the muscle cells, where it can be burned off and used as an energy source. If your blood sugar level is high, you secrete a lot of insulin. If your blood sugar level is low, you secrete less insulin.

Your blood sugar level rises when you eat simple sugars and certain carbohydrate foods. In fact, eating lots of certain carbohydrates—like white flour and potatoes—and sugars causes a sharp increase in your blood sugar level. This surge is what gives an energy rush, or "sugar high." You know the feeling you get when you eat a big candy bar at one sitting? Hyper, then somewhat sleepy? Well, when blood sugar levels are quickly elevated to a high level, the pancreas secretes a lot of insulin right away—more insulin than is necessary to balance the blood sugar.

Some people, after a sharp rise in blood sugar levels, may experience a "rebound" reaction where their blood sugar is lowered even below its starting point. That's when they'll feel a letdown, or "sugar low." They may feel tired, listless, and artificially hungry. They may feel like taking a nap. Or, they'll reach for something sweet or caffeinated to give them more energy. Then the cycle repeats itself! The sugar goes in, the blood sugar goes up, the pancreas secretes insulin, the blood sugar drops below normal, and they'll feel tired and hungry again. This vicious cycle causes some people to eat more and more empty sugar calories without ever satisfying their nutritional needs.

Does this sound familiar? A wonderful woman on the set of my television show *Step by Step*, named Inger, makes fantastic meals for us, so we don't have to take time out of the day to have lunch outside the studio. Well, before I started Somersizing, every day at three, my energy level would begin to drop due to a poorly combined lunch. Inger would bring me some hot, fresh-baked chocolate chip cookies, which I'd devour. I'd feel great—for a short while. I eventually developed a Pavlovian response; every day at three, my body would know it was "cookie time." When I started Somersizing, though, I lost my sugar craving. I had never before in my life turned down a cookie, but when Inger brought them to me, I simply didn't want them anymore.

Energy level highs and lows cause us to eat way more than our appetites require. The reason we feel artificially hungry is that the extra insulin in the blood inhibits the body from producing another hormone, serotonin, which is what makes the brain realize that the stomach is full. Your brain thinks, Too much insulin? Not enough fuel in the blood. We need to eat! *The foods you eat may contain more energy than you need. And excess energy that isn't burned off is stored as fat for later use.* (Of course, your activity level determines that quotient. More on this in Chapter 8.)

Think about how many carbohydrates you eat in a normal day and compare that with how much your body actually needs for fuel. Unless you're a marathon runner, you're probably storing an ample supply of fat reserves from overindulging in simple sugars and certain carbohydrates. This Irish girl's heart once sank at the thought of giving up potatoes. But when I think now about the *kind* and *amount* of carbos I used to eat, as well as how I combined my foods, I understand why I gained weight.

Here's the really important part. When the body needs energy, the first source it will think to look at for fuel is carbohydrates. And guess what? If there's no sugar and highly starchy foods to turn to for quick energy sources, the body has to look elsewhere for vital energy. Guess where the body looks first? Your fat reserves! Fat reserves are the body's vital energy source. That layer of fat starts melting away as you are infused with energy, all the while eating delicious, nutritious foods loaded with flavor. You can actually force your body to use your fat reserves as an energy source by eliminating sugar and high-starch foods.

That's the key to Somersizing: to convert your body from a carbo-burning machine into a fat-burning machine.

By limiting your intake of sugars and

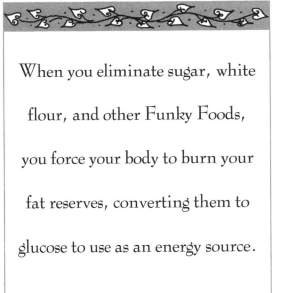

When you eliminate sugar, white flour, and other Funky Foods, you force your body to burn your fat reserves, converting them to glucose to use as an energy source.

starches, you force your body to dip into its fat reserves as a source of energy. Fat is one of the most highly concentrated forms of food energy. Imagine the burning of a candle, made from animal fat, and what happens when you burn a piece of toast. That toast just burns right up, and then the flame is out. Fat is an even source of energy to get you through the day, without sugar highs and lows. When you Somersize, your energy level remains constant. You'll be surprised at how much and the variety of foods you can eat because you are giving your body good, nutritious foods that appease your appetite. You eat until you are satisfied and comfortable, period.

Carbohydrates in a refined form are much harder on the body than those in a natural form. In the last century, we have refined most of the nutrients out of our foods. Who was it that decided rice would be better without its nutty brown shell? Brown rice has a wonderful flavor and is loaded with fiber you won't find in refined white rice. And how about white flour? Breads and pastas used to be made with natural whole grains. As grains became more refined, we as a society gained more and more weight. Since our average American diet is made up of lots of refined carbohydrates like sugar, white flour, white-flour pasta, and instant potatoes, it's no wonder obesity is epidemic in our country!

Being thin is not just a vanity issue. It is cause for great concern regarding one's general health. Obesity is a risk factor that contributes to diseases leading to premature death—right up there with cigarette smoking. Please, do yourself, do your body, and do your loved ones a favor and stop filling up on empty carbohydrates that leave you nutritionally unsatisfied, overweight, and even emotionally unstable.

Now, I know what some of you are thinking: How can some friends live on junk food, like candy bars and cheeseburgers with french fries, and be thin as a rail? The answer is that each of us is created differently, with a unique and ever-changing metabolism. Some people have perfect metabolisms that always burn the food they eat as fuel, rather than storing it as fat. They have a pancreas that always secretes the proper amount of insulin to balance their blood sugar, regardless of what they eat. For the record, we hate these people (just kidding). Other people, like myself, may start out with a perfect metabolism, but find as they get older that their metabolism has changed and they must work to avoid a weight problem.

My nephew Russell has been fighting his weight problem all his life. He's tried everything, including starving himself. He's one of those people born with an unfortunately low metabolism. Somersizing has changed

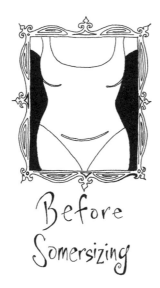

Before
Somersizing

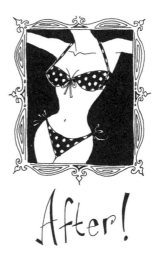

After!

his life. He's lost so much weight that his whole office is now on the program. His wife says, "Everything is better since he lost weight. He's so much happier with himself now that he looks and feels more attractive." It worked for Russell; it can work for you, too.

How we combine the foods we eat can lead to weight gain and digestive problems. Eating proteins and carbohydrates together puts a strain on the digestive process because these two groups of foods are broken down by different digestive enzymes. Proteins, like meat, are used by the body to build muscle tissue. To be broken down and metabolized, protein requires an acidic environment. Carbohydrates, like bread, are used by the body as a quick energy source. To be broken down and metabolized, carbohydrates require a basic environment that's the opposite of the acidic conditions required for protein metabolism.

When you eat a poorly combined meal of meat with bread, the acid from the protein and the base from the bread can lead to a halt in the digestive process. During this delay in digestion, bacteria in the food can begin to ferment, creating gas and bloating, which is why you may feel very uncomfortable after a big meal. A common reason for gas and bloating is a poorly combined meal. And in this slowed-down digestive process, there is more opportunity for food to be stored as fat, rather than burned off and used as fuel. (Gas can also stem from lactose intolerance, mental or physical stress, or a diet too high in fiber without enough water intake. Excessive gas can come from swallowing air while eating or

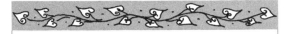

When you eat in proper Somersized combinations, you are helping your body digest food more quickly and efficiently.

drinking, and even from eating "gas-forming" vegetables like beans, broccoli, brussels sprouts, cabbage, lentils, cucumbers, apples, and avocados.)

Then there's the question of energy level. Our bodies expend a tremendous amount of energy in digesting food. Not only will a poorly combined meal leave you gassy and bloated but it will leave you tired because it requires the body to put even more energy into digestion. Your vital energy is being zapped for digestion.

Somersizing solves all of these problems. Proteins and carbohydrates are eaten separately and combined only with vegetables, which can be broken down by either an acid or a base environment. And fruit is eaten alone, on an empty stomach, which allows for smooth digestion, as you'll learn later.

Whenever I get a chance, I go to Tuscany to enjoy the foods of the region. I'm always struck by the fact that, after a big meal of pasta and vegetables and soup and meat and wine, the Tuscan natives bring out a tray of fruit. They've had such a heavy meal, they want to eat something nice and light and sweet. So it was no surprise when one day I walked into a local pharmacy, in a tiny village called Radda, in Chianti, to see an entire wall devoted to antacids! These people must lie awake all night with horrible stomach pain after their fruit desserts.

The good news is that by Somersizing, you don't have to say good-bye to sugar and starches forever. Soon you will be down to your goal weight and you can begin Level Two, where you incorporate some sugar and starches in moderation without gaining back the weight. Every now and then I have to have a little chocolate . . . so I have it. But I make sure it's really worth it.

Now that you understand why Somersizing works, let's take a look at exactly how you'll be eating in order to look and feel your best. The next section will show you what foods to eliminate so as to aid in digestion and weight control.

CHAPTER FOUR

Eliminate the Funky Foods

SUGAR, WHITE FLOUR, AND FUNKY FOODS

As you've learned, all the food you eat every day can be divided into four Somersize groups: Proteins and Fats, Vegetables, Carbohydrates, and Fruits. The fifth group is the one you'll be eliminating from your diet entirely. This is a group of foods that causes your blood sugar to rise rapidly. I call these Funky Foods. There are four basic kinds.

The first kind of Funky Foods are sugar sources. Even though some of these are in their natural form, they're still sugar, so avoid them completely when trying to lose weight.

SUGARS
White sugar
Brown sugar
Raw sugar
Corn syrup

Sucrose
Fructose
Molasses
Honey
Maple syrup
Beets
Carrots

I know it seems weird to eliminate carrots, which have many good nutritional qualities, including essential beta-carotene and vitamin A. But carrots are very high in carbohydrates (or natural sugar) and there's plenty of beta-carotene in apricots (dried and raw), cantaloupe, collard greens, broccoli, and kale, which you can eat in abundance. Vitamin A is found in cantaloupe, peaches, and apricots. With regard to sugar, honey, and maple syrup, if I find I must have something sweet, I use artificial sweeteners like Equal or Sweet 'N Low.

Read food labels carefully. Fructose—

fruit sugar—is often in products labeled "healthy" or "dietetic." And believe it or not, sugar is often added to products such as prepared tomato pastes and sauces.

The second kind of Funky Foods are those high in starch. These foods turn directly to sugar (glucose) in our bodies upon digestion. Remember, you don't need to give your body extra sugar because you want to encourage it to use your fat reserves for energy.

STARCHES
White or Semolina flour
Pasta or couscous (made from
semolina or white flour)
White rice
Corn/popcorn
Potatoes, sweet potatoes, or yams
Pumpkin
Winter squashes (butternut, acorn)
Bananas

There are so many wonderful alternatives to white flour and semolina. Look for breads and pastas made from whole wheat, rye, amaranth, spelt, and kamut, to name a few. Replace white rice with brown rice, which has a wonderful nutty, earthy flavor. Better yet, try wild rice, which contains even less starch. As for corn and potatoes, you will be eating greater amounts of green vegetables rather than filling up on starchy vegetables, which cause a sugar surge and add pounds. Think about this: corn and potatoes are what's most often used to fatten our livestock. Now, maybe you won't find it so hard to resist that plate of fries!

"What's wrong with bananas?" you ask. "They're loaded with potassium!" Sorry, but bananas are also very high in starch. With all the other fruits you *can* eat, you won't miss them. You can also get potassium from mangoes, celery, broccoli, tomatoes, prunes, oranges, lemons, and asparagus.

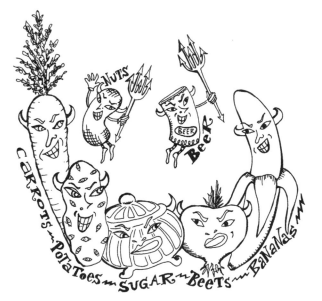

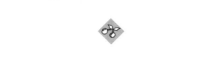

Jean Pierre Fougeirol, who told me all about food combining.

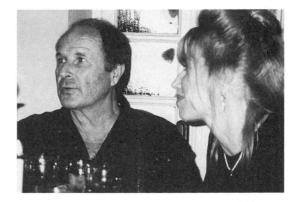

WHAT TO DRINK?

Well, if you're cutting out caffeinated soda and coffee, what should *you drink?*

Water. I highly recommend you drink eight to ten glasses of water a day (more for those who exercise or live in a hot environment). You can also have Crystal Light–type drinks sweetened with NutraSweet, decaffeinated coffee, teas, and even sodas. (Personally, I stay away from diet and soft drinks because they are loaded with chemicals. You would be doing your body a favor to eliminate them as well.)

Another Somersize tip: Try not to drink with your *meals because water can dilute your digestive juices, which slows down the digestive process. If you must drink with your meal, eat a portion of your food before you drink anything.*

The third kind of Funky Foods don't fit neatly into one of the four Somersize Food Groups because these foods contain both protein and/or fat *and* carbohydrates. For example, consider low-fat or whole milk. Either has protein, fat, and carbohydrates, which make it a no-no for Somersizing purposes. (Nonfat dairy products are grouped as Carbohydrates.)

BAD COMBO FOODS
Nuts
Olives
Liver
Avocados
Coconuts
Low-fat or whole milk
Tofu and soy milk

If you are a vegan or strict vegetarian, I do make an exception regarding tofu and soy milk as additional protein sources. Although tofu has protein, fat, and carbohydrates, treat it as a Proteins/Fats and combine it only with Veggies. Reduced-fat tofu is acceptable as a Proteins/Fats. Also, try using textured soy protein. It comes in a zillion forms—shaped into burgers or frank-furters, or crumbled to resemble ground beef, for use in tacos, chilis, and other dishes. Look for those products that contain only textured soy protein—no grain filler.

The last kind of Funky Foods are caffeine and alcohol. Caffeinated coffees, teas, and cocoas are stimulants. Feel free to drink decaffeinated coffee and herbal teas. When you combine your foods correctly, you'll get a natural energy boost instead of an artificial caffeine buzz.

As for alcohol, everyone knows it can make you fat (especially beer and hard liquor). Even though alcohol contains no fat, it is a carbohydrate that your body tends to store immediately as fat. Alcohol contains very few nutrients and is a depressant. When you're drinking alcohol, you may not make the wisest food choices. Red wine has recently been found to have some health benefits, and can be incorporated in moder-ation in Level Two. But during Level One, steer clear of all alcohol, except in cooking, where it burns off but leaves its flavor behind.

CAFFEINE AND ALCOHOL
Coffee
Caffeinated teas
Caffeinated sodas
Cocoa
Beer
Hard alcohol
Wine

Eliminating these foods will soon become second nature to you. Sugar, starches, bad combo foods, caffeine, and alcohol are all avoided on Level One. But don't worry, you don't have to say good-bye to these foods forever. They'll be back in moderation when you reach your goal weight and begin main-taining it on Level Two.

CHAPTER FIVE

Separate . . .

You know all about what *not* to eat. Now the second—and best!—key to Somersizing is all the delicious foods you *can* eat. In this chapter, I show you how to separate foods into the components of healthy meals that will stimulate your metabolism. Here are those key Somersize Food Groups.

PROTEINS/FATS

This group is made up of foods high in protein and/or fat. Many of the foods that contain protein also contain fat, and so I've combined these nutrients into one group. You can eat any of the foods in this group together or in combination with Veggies.

Proteins are made up of organic compounds called amino acids. Amino acids are the building blocks of the human body, necessary for cell growth. They play a role in virtually every cellular function, from regulating muscle contraction, antibody production, and blood vessel expansion and contraction, to maintaining normal blood pressure. Protein is a critically important part of the human diet. The human body cannot produce protein on its own; it can derive it only from dietary sources.

As far as fat is concerned, it is true that a diet too high in fats can contribute to health problems. But eliminating fat completely from your diet is unhealthy, too. Fats are a major source of stored metabolic fuel. They break down to provide energy and help facilitate the use of essential fat-soluble vitamins like A, D, E, and K. Vitamin A is necessary for healthy eyes and skin; vitamin D helps to metabolize calcium; vitamin E prevents cholesterol deposits; and vitamin K contributes to healthy blood clotting. Essential fatty acids supplied by fats cannot be manufactured by our bodies on their own; they, too, must be included in our daily meals.

Fats can come in three forms—saturated, unsaturated, and monounsaturated (olive and canola oils). Saturated fats, such as those found in meat, cheese, and butter, can increase cholesterol levels, so eat these fats in moderation. However, unsaturated fats, like corn oil, safflower oil, or soy bean oil, actually help lower cholesterol levels and can be included in your meals to a reasonable degree.

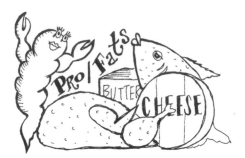

The following are Proteins/Fats:

CHEESE

American	Colby	Jarlsberg	Provolone
Asiago	Farmer	Limburger	Queso blanco
Babybel	Feta	Mascarpone	Ricotta
Bel Paese	Fontina	Monterey Jack	Romano
Blue	Goat	Mozzarella	Roquefort
Bonbel	Gouda	Mozzarella, buffalo	String
Brie	Gruyère	Muenster	Swiss
Camembert	Havarti	Parmesan	
Cheddar	Hoop	Pecorino	

OTHER DAIRY PRODUCTS

Butter	Eggs	Mayonnaise
Cream	Margarine	Sour cream

FISH

Anchovies	Flounder	Orange roughy	Snapper
Bass	Gefilte fish	Pollock	Sole
Bluefish	Grouper	Pompano	Sturgeon
Bonito	Haddock	Red snapper	Swordfish
Burbot	Halibut	Sablefish	Trout
Carp	Herring	Salmon	Tuna
Catfish	Mackerel	Sardines	Turbot
Cod	Mahimahi	Sea bass	Whitefish
Eel	Monkfish	Shark	Wolf fish
Flat fish	Ocean perch	Smelt	Yellowtail

MEAT

Bacon	Frogs' legs	Pepperoni	Sausage
Beef	Ham	Pork	Veal
Bockwurst	Hot dogs	Prosciutto	Venison
Canadian bacon	Lamb	Rabbit	
Cold cuts	Pastrami	Salami	

OILS

Chili oil	Olive oil	Sesame oil	Vegetable oil
Corn oil	Safflower oil	Peanut oil	

POULTRY

Capon	Duck	Guinea hen	Quail
Chicken	Goose	Pheasant	Squab
Cornish hen			

SEAFOOD

Abalone	Crab	Mussels	Shrimp
Caviar	Crayfish	Octopus	Squid
Clams	Lobster	Scallops	

Note: If you are a vegetarian and find you are not getting enough protein, you may include tofu and soy milk in your Proteins/Fats meals. Tofu is a Funky Food made from soybeans, which contain very high amounts of protein plus fat and carbohydrates, but I make an exception for strict vegetarians.

CARBOS

Carbohydrates are derived from plant rather than animal sources. They are the primary metabolic fuel in our modern Western diets. Carbohydrates break down into glucose, which is the body's main source of energy. I divide carbohydrates into two categories: refined and complex. You'll find refined carbohydrates like sugar and white flour in the Funky Foods group. These foods are to be avoided completely in Level One. You can, however, enjoy complex carbohydrates, such as whole-grain breads, to your heart's content. Complex carbohydrates contain essential vitamins and nutrients and provide fiber necessary for the digestive process.

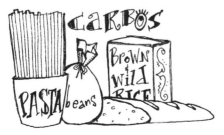

Unlike refined carbohydrates, complex carbos do not provoke a sudden spike in insulin levels. They are broken down more slowly in your system. You can eat any of the foods in this group together, or in combination with Veggies. Both beans and nonfat dairy products are sources of protein. But because of the way your body reacts to them and because they're high in carbohydrates as well, I've put them in the Carbohydrate group.

BEANS

Adzuki	Cannellini (white)	Lentils	Peas, green
Anasazi	Fava (broad)	Lima	Pinto
Black (turtle)	Garbanzo (chickpeas)	Mung	Red
Black-eyed peas	Kidney	Navy	Split peas

BREADS, BAGELS, CRACKERS, HOT CEREALS, COLD CEREALS, PASTA, RICE, OR PHYLLO DOUGH MADE FROM WHOLE GRAINS

Amaranth	Buckwheat	Oats	Wheat
Barley	Bulgur	Rye	Wheat germ
Bran	Kamut	Spelt	Wild rice
Brown rice	Millet		

MUSTARD

Brown	Dijon	Whole-grain	Yellow

NONFAT DAIRY PRODUCTS

Cheeses	Cream cheese	Sour cream
Cottage cheese	Milk	Yogurt

There are some foods I consider "tricky," like sun-dried tomatoes. These are Veggies, but they tend to be packed in oil, so you can use them only in a Proteins/Fats meal, not in a Carbos meal. Sometimes you can find dry (no-oil) sun-dried tomatoes, which would be okay with Carbos. The same goes for mushrooms and artichoke hearts marinated in oil. Always be certain to check the ingredients list. Finally, botanically speaking, tomatoes are fruit. But their sugar content is closer to that of vegetables, and because they behave in your system more like Veggies than Fruits, that's the group in which I've put them. The other exceptions to the Fruits rule are low-sugar lemons and limes, which can be used as a garnish or for flavor with any food, at any time. Soy sauce, vinegar, and spices are also okay to use with any of the four food groups.

VEGGIES

Vegetables are technically carbohydrates, but because the vegetables I've selected cause only a minute rise in your blood sugar, they deserve their own Somersized category. You can eat Veggies alone, or with Proteins/Fats or Carbos.

Vegetables are packed with nutrients and provide essential roughage for proper elimination.

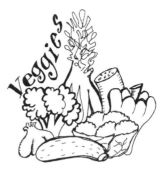

Alfalfa sprouts
Artichokes
Arugula
Asparagus
Bamboo shoots
Basil
Bean sprouts
Beet greens
Bok choy
Broccoli
Brussels sprouts
Cabbage
Cauliflower
Celery
Chervil
Chicory
Chives
Cilantro
Clover sprouts
Collard greens
Crookneck squash
Cucumber
Daikon
Dandelion greens
Dill
Eggplant
Endive

Escarole
Fennel
Garlic
Ginger
Green beans
Horseradish
Kale
Kohlrabi
Leeks
Lettuce
    Boston or Bibb
    Iceberg
    Limestone
    Red oak leaf
    Romaine
Mushrooms
Mustard greens
Okra
Onions
Parsley
Parsnips
Peppers
    Bell peppers
    Cherry peppers
    Chili peppers
    Peperoncini
    Piccalilli

Pickles
    (except sweet)
Purslane
Radicchio
Radishes
Rhubarb
Rosemary
Sage
Salsify
Sauerkraut
Shallots
Snow peas
Spinach
Sugar snap peas
Swiss chard
Tarragon
Thyme
Tomatillo
Tomato
Tomato, green
Turnip
Turnip greens
Watercress
Wax beans
Yard-long beans
Yellow beans
Zucchini

Like vegetables, fruits are also technically carbohydrates. But because of their sugar content, fruit must always be eaten alone. Fruits are a great source of fiber, and they help keep the digestive tract working properly. They are loaded with nutrients and vitamins. But if you mix fruits with other foods, they can lose their nutritional benefits and upset the digestive process.

Fruit turns to acid when combined with other food groups and spoils in the stomach, causing gas pain, pressure, and that horrible bloated feeling. Fruit as a supposedly "healthy" dessert option can ruin a perfectly combined meal. Remember "zee cherries!"

So eat fruit . . . *please* eat fruit. But eat it on an empty stomach. You can have it first thing in the morning, or wait two hours after your last meal to have it as a snack or dessert.

You can also eat fruit alone, then wait twenty minutes and have a Carbohydrates meal. Or eat fruit alone, wait an hour, and have a Proteins/Fats meal. The only exception to all of this is that I've found you can use the juice of lemons and limes to add flavor to Proteins/Fats, Carbos, or Veggies because they are very low in sugar and do not upset the digestive process of other foods.

Apple
Apricot
Asian pear
Berries
   Blackberry
   Blueberry
   Boysenberry
   Cranberry
   Currant
   Elderberry
   Gooseberry
   Mulberry
   Ollalaberry
   Raspberry
   Strawberry

Cherimoya
Cherries
Crabapple
Fig
Grapefruit
Grapes
Guava
Kiwi
Kumquat
Lemon
Lime
Loquat
Mandarin oranges

Mango
Melon
   Cantaloupe
   Cassava
   Crenshaw
   Honeydew
   Orange flesh
   Sharlyn
   Watermelon
Nectarine
Orange
Papaya
Passion fruit

Peach
Pear
Persimmon
Pineapple
Plum
Pomegranate
Pomelo
Prickly pear
Quince
Star fruit
Tamarind
Tangelo
Tangerine

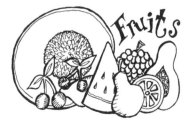

CHAPTER SIX

✧

. . . And Somersize!

Now that you have a basic understanding of what foods to eliminate and how to categorize the rest of the foods you eat into four Somersize Food Groups, you can get started on your new lifestyle. Once again, here are the seven easy steps for combining foods to get the most nutritional value, without digestive difficulties like bloating or gas.

1. Eliminate all Funky Foods.
2. Eat Fruits alone, on an empty stomach.
3. Eat Proteins/Fats with Veggies.
4. Eat Carbos with Veggies and no fat.
5. Keep Proteins/Fats separate from Carbos.
6. Wait three hours between meals if switching from a Proteins/Fats meal to a Carbos meal, or vice versa.
7. Do not skip meals. Eat three meals a day, and eat until you feel satisfied and comfortably full.

Any of the foods in the Proteins/Fats group can be eaten together, or in combination with Veggies.

Any of the foods in the Carbos group can be eaten together, or in combination with Veggies.

Any of the foods in the Veggies group can be eaten together. And since Veggies can easily be digested with either Proteins/Fats or Carbos, you can eat them with either group.

Any of the foods in the Fruits group can be eaten together. But there are some guidelines to follow when eating fruit:

- Eat Fruits on an empty stomach.
- Eat Fruits alone, then wait 20 minutes and follow up with a Carbos meal. (The 20-minute lead time gets the digestion of the fruit going and eliminates problem combinations.)
- Eat Fruits alone, then wait one hour and follow up with a Proteins/Fats meal.

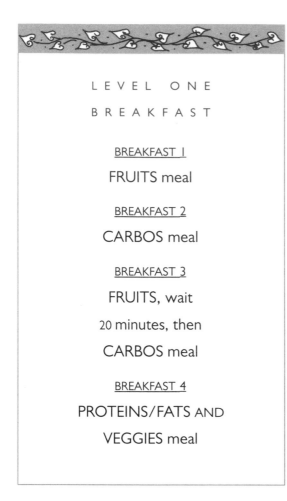

combinations, you can eat *any* of those foods for breakfast—just not in the same sitting.

All the foods listed below make up perfectly combined Somersize breakfasts, so you may eat until you are satisfied and comfortably full.

BREAKFAST 1— FRUITS MEAL

Start your day off with an apple, a couple of tangelos, or some melon. Create a Fruit Smoothie (page 88) in your blender with any of your favorite fruits, a little fruit juice, and a few ice cubes. Make a fruit salad and dig in. You can eat any kind of fruit except bananas, which are a Funky Food. Fruit is best in the morning, when you eat it on an empty stomach. Try any of these:

- Fruit Smoothie with raspberries, strawberries, blackberries, and a little fruit juice
- Fruit Smoothie with unsweetened pineapple chunks, papaya, and orange juice
- Fruit salad of melon, grapes, apples, and oranges
- Pears, mangoes, or melon

To drink, have decaf coffee or decaf tea, with artificial sweetener, if desired.

- If you want fruit for a snack or for dessert, you must wait two hours after your last meal to avoid any problems.

At every meal, you get to decide what you want to eat. Whether you're eating at home or at a restaurant, your choices are endless.

Let's go through all three meals, starting with the first one of the day. What do you like to eat for breakfast—cereal, toast, fruit, eggs, bacon, sausage? How about all of them? As long as you follow the Somersize

BREAKFAST 2— CARBOS MEAL

I love to eat Carbos in the morning! There are a number of wonderful options. I like whole-grain toast with nonfat cottage cheese or yogurt. Or I have hot or cold cereal with nonfat milk. (Remember, you can have Veggies with your Carbos, so feel free to top your toast with tomatoes or a slice of red onion, if you like. No jelly!) To get you started thinking:

- Whole wheat toast with nonfat cottage cheese
- Pumpernickel bagel with nonfat ricotta cheese
- Rye bagel with nonfat cream cheese, tomatoes, and onion
- Fat-free wheat tortilla with black beans, tomatoes, and enchilada sauce
- Grape-Nuts cereal with nonfat yogurt
- Shredded wheat with nonfat milk
- Oatmeal with nonfat milk

To drink, have decaf coffee or tea with nonfat milk and/or artificial sweetener.

BREAKFAST 3 — FRUITS, THEN CARBOS MEAL

Fruits then Carbos is my favorite choice for breakfast because these foods provide me with necessary fiber and a whole host of vitamins and nutrients. Besides that, they just taste good! Alan is the master breakfast maker in our home. Usually he brings me a great Fruit Smoothie in the morning. Then I have my bath and get ready for work. Afterward we have toast or cereal with decaf coffee. Morning is the best time to eat your Fruits and Carbos so that you have plenty of time to burn off the energy they provide.

Here are a few more examples of breakfasts:

- Melon; wait 20 minutes, then Cream of Wheat cereal with nonfat milk
- Fruit Smoothie with peaches, strawberries, and orange juice; wait 20 minutes, then whole-grain toast with nonfat cottage cheese and a sprinkle of cinnamon
- A couple of tangerines; wait 20 minutes, then Puffed Wheat cereal with nonfat milk
- Pineapple juice; wait 20 minutes, then toasted rye bagel with nonfat cream cheese
- Fruit salad; wait 20 minutes, then oatmeal with nonfat milk

To drink, have decaf coffee or tea with nonfat milk and/or artificial sweetener.

BREAKFAST 4 — PROTEINS/ FATS AND VEGGIES MEAL

In a Proteins/Fats and Veggies breakfast, you can have anything from the Proteins/Fats group with anything from the Veggies group. The options are limitless. Have eggs scrambled, fried, boiled, poached, or made into an omelet or a frittata. Cook them in butter, margarine, or oil. Enjoy meats, fish, and poultry like bacon, sausage, turkey, chicken, shrimp, crab, and smoked fish. Top it off with any kind of cheese you like, and don't forget to add Veggies like onions, tomatoes, zucchini, spinach, mushrooms, and asparagus.

This is a great breakfast option when

you're eating out because there are so few restrictions. Just stay away from toast, potatoes, and fruit. And make smart choices when it comes to breakfast foods that are high in saturated fats, like bacon, ham, and sausage. Although you may eat these foods, you should limit your intake in order to keep your cholesterol under control. I choose lean meats when I have a Protein/Fat breakfast, and if I find I'm eating too many eggs, I use only the egg whites. Try one of these:

- Omelet with spinach, cheese, and mushrooms; side of turkey sausage
- Fried eggs with bacon or sausage; side of tomatoes
- Scrambled eggs with smoked salmon, sour cream, and green onions; side of zucchini
- Poached eggs with Canadian bacon; side of asparagus
- Egg white omelet with bell peppers, onions, and mushrooms; side of broccoli

To drink, have decaf coffee or tea with cream and/or artificial sweetener.

(*Note:* If you want to start this meal with Fruits, you must wait one hour until you have your Proteins/Fats and Veggies.)

Okay, let's move on to lunch and dinner. What do you like to eat—salads, soups, sandwiches, chicken, steak, or pasta? All of these foods are okay if eaten in proper combinations. First you have to decide what food group you feel like having.

Many of these are my own favorite recipes, which you'll find in the next few chapters.

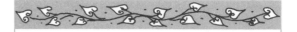

LEVEL ONE
LUNCH OR DINNER

LUNCH OR DINNER 1
CARBOS and VEGGIES meal

LUNCH OR DINNER 2
PROTEINS/FATS and
VEGGIES meal

LUNCH OR DINNER 3
SINGLE FOOD GROUP meal

LUNCH OR DINNER 1— CARBOS AND VEGGIES MEAL

If you feel like Carbos and Veggies, you might have Black Bean Chili with Spicy Tomato Salsa (page 143) and whole wheat tortillas or a whole-grain pasta with Simple Tomato, Basil, and Garlic Sauce (page 145) and a green salad, or pitas with Baba Ganoush (page 75), Hummus (page 77), and fresh vegetables. The key to this meal is to make sure there is no fat. (Even foods like beans and vegetables contain a tiny trace of fat. So whenever I say "fat-free," or "nonfat," I mean that there's less than ½ gram of fat per serving. For Somersizing purposes, this small amount of fat is inconsequential.)

All the whole grains and vegetables make this a satisfying and healthy option. But it can be a little restrictive because you can't have added fat and you must watch for hidden sugars and Funky Foods on Level One. Take a look at my nonfat sandwich spread and soup recipes in Chapter 11. And there are a few good nonfat cheeses on the market that are perfectly okay to use in your Carbos and Veggies Meals. This meal is more difficult when you're eating in a restaurant. I normally prepare Carbos and Veggies meals, like the following, at home.

- Vegetarian sandwich made with whole-grain bread, lettuce, tomato, pickles, onions, peppers, sprouts, and mustard; green salad with fat-free dressing
- Whole wheat pitas with nonfat ricotta cheese, Roasted Red Peppers (page 81), and Grilled Eggplant (page 90); green salad with fat-free dressing

Somersizing allows you to relax and enjoy meals and good conversation without guilt and deprivation.

- Penne with Simple Tomato, Basil, and Garlic Sauce (page 145) and a whole-grain roll
- Roasted Red Pepper Soup (page 131); brown rice with steamed vegetables, seasoned with soy sauce and red pepper flakes
- Whole wheat tortilla with nonfat cheese, tomatoes, pinto beans, and salsa; green salad with fat-free dressing
- Whole wheat pita with Hummus (page 77), Baba Ganoush (page 75), lettuce, and tomato; Cold Cucumber Asparagus Soup (page 134)
- Spinach pasta with garden vegetables and stewed tomatoes; fresh raw vegetables with Cannellini Bean Dip (page 74)
- Whole Wheat Cheeseless Pizza (page 142); green salad with fat-free dressing
- Black Bean Chili with Spicy Tomato Salsa (page 143) and whole wheat tortillas; green salad with fat-free dressing

To drink, have water, mineral water, decaf coffee, or tea with nonfat milk and/or artificial sweetener.

LUNCH OR DINNER 2 — PROTEINS/FATS AND VEGGIES MEAL

You can order with ease from any restaurant menu with the Proteins/Fats and Veggies meal. Meat, poultry, or fish can be grilled, broiled, baked, roasted, or fried and served with plenty of fresh vegetables, raw, steamed, sautéed, or grilled. Most good restaurants do not add sugar to their sauces and salad dressings, so you may enjoy them to the fullest. If the dressings *do* have sugar, it's the easiest thing in the world to ask for the oil and vinegar cruets instead.

Enjoy cooking with oil or butter and don't forget to add the cheese! But I do caution you to manage your intake of foods high in saturated fats. If you had a bacon cheeseburger for lunch (without the bun), consider going lighter on the dinner menu.

You will have no problem creating wonderful Proteins/Fats and Veggies meals. With so much to choose from, you won't ever get bored eating the same old thing. Here are some of my favorite recipes:

- Cobb salad of sliced chicken, bacon, egg, tomato, blue cheese, and green onions with Italian dressing
- Taco Salad of shredded beef, tomatoes, Cheddar cheese, salsa, onions, and sour cream (page 122)
- Chicken Tomato Cilantro Soup (page 126); green salad with dressing of your choice
- Fillet of Sole with Lemon Caper Butter and Seared Spinach (page 152); raw vegetables with onion dip
- Grilled Chicken Caesar Salad (page 117)
- Turkey burger patty with melted jack cheese; sautéed vegetables with a sprinkle of Parmesan cheese
- Broccoli Leek Soup (page 133)
- Tuna Salad in Lettuce Cups (page 119), with tomato slices and alfalfa sprouts

- Roasted chicken (page 164); Crunchy Cabbage Salad with red wine vinaigrette (page 110); steamed broccoli and zucchini
- Green salad with fresh crabmeat and dressing of your choice
- Grilled Pepper Steak with Herb Butter (page 174); steamed asparagus
- Steamed Artichokes with Lemon-Dill Mayonnaise (page 85)
- Turkey Cutlet with Classic Marinara Sauce (page 170); Greek Salad (page 113)
- Grilled Lamb Chops with Fresh Herbs (page 177); Vegetables Provençal (page 92)
- Chicken with stir-fried vegetables
- Chopped Salami and Vegetable Salad (page 114)

To drink, have water, mineral water, decaf coffee, or tea with cream and/or artificial sweetener.

LUNCH OR DINNER 3 — SINGLE FOOD GROUP MEAL

Every now and then you might want to have a meal made up of only one food group, like the all-Fruits meal or the all-Veggies meal. Of course, this is perfectly fine. This option includes those meals where you want just a simple fruit salad or a plate of steamed vegetables.

CHAPTER SEVEN

The Top Ten Somersize Questions

A few months ago, my nephew Russell had just started the Somersize program, and asked me, "Can you eat meat with beans?" As I answered him with a resounding "No!" I realized that what has become second nature to me—no, you can't eat Proteins and Fats (meat) with Carbos (beans)—takes newcomers a little while to understand. So here are the top ten most common Somersize questions.

1. Should I eat more Proteins/Fats meals or Carbos meals?

Even though I always stress that you can choose to have either Carbos or Proteins/Fats at every meal, people often ask me if it's better to choose one over the other. In general, I find that the fewer carbohydrates I eat, the more weight I lose. Carbohydrates are an energy source, and if you're not giving your body any sources of energy, it has no choice but to break down your fat

reserves for energy. But it's important to incorporate some Carbos because they have a lot of good fiber and help keep your system moving properly. I like to have a Fruits, then Carbos breakfast, and there are so many great choices. For lunch or dinner I find more options with Proteins/Fats and plenty of Veggies. Carbos meals for lunch and dinner are a little more restrictive because you can have absolutely no fat.

My recommendation is that for breakfast you usually have Breakfast 3—Fruits, then Carbos. For lunch, choose either Lunch 1—Carbos and Veggies—or Lunch 2—Proteins/Fats and Veggies. At dinner you're probably better off having Dinner 2—Proteins/Fats and Veggies—because you don't need the energy from carbohydrates that late in the day, and if you regularly eat carbohydrates at night and don't use the energy, they could get stored as fat for later use.

This is only a blueprint of how I divide

my Proteins/Fats and Carbos meals—you may find that your body can handle more carbohydrates and that you feel better eating mostly grains and vegetables. For me, those carbohydrates tend to stick to my hips when I eat them too often. On the other hand, if you are eating mostly Proteins/Fats meals, make sure to round them out with plenty of fresh vegetables. Watch your fat intake, and don't get excessive with the protein you eat because too much can be hard on your system.

2. I can eat fat and still lose weight? This sounds too good to be true.

As long as you are properly combining, you can eat moderate amounts of fat and still lose weight. When you combine fats with carbohydrates, it can upset your digestive system. For instance, if I ate a grilled ham and cheese sandwich, I would feel bloated and uncomfortable. But if I ate the ham and cheese without the bread—with some fresh grilled vegetables, for example—I would feel satisfied and healthy.

How about cholesterol? Foods of animal origin—such as meats and butters—are generally high in cholesterol, and should be eaten in moderation; that's common sense. I know one person who heard about Somersizing from a friend, but didn't understand the whole program. Some of the meals he ate consisted of six eggs, half a pound of bacon, and a side of broccoli smothered in cheese sauce. He was very careful not to eat any carbohydrates with these meals, and he lost eighteen pounds in six weeks! Yes, you *can* eat fat and still lose weight as long as you are not combining with any carbohydrates.

But this guy's cholesterol level increased by fifty points! This is not a smart way to Somersize. I do not recommend you eat this way. Choose lean meats, fresh fish, and unsaturated oils that actually help lower your cholesterol.

3. How should I order when I eat out at a restaurant?

I realize this information may seem a bit overwhelming at first, but soon you will discover how simple Somersizing can be. So many people tell me, "I eat two out of three of my meals each day in restaurants; it's impossible to lose weight." Once you understand Somersizing, eating in a restaurant is truly easy.

First I scan the menu and decide if I want a Proteins/Fats and Veggies meal or a Carbos and Veggies meal. A Proteins/Fats meal might be chicken piccata with a lovely lemon and caper butter sauce; steamed, sautéed, or grilled vegetables; and a green salad with my choice of dressing. A Carbos and Veggies meal might be a vegetarian sandwich on whole-grain bread or brown rice with steamed vegetables and soy sauce.

The key to the Proteins/Fats meal is *no* bread, pasta, potatoes, or rice. These are the things that throw your system into chaos. You'll be surprised at how quickly you'll get over missing the starch. Some quick tips:

- Pass the bread basket to someone across the table and leave it there.
- Watch for hidden sugars or starches in the salad dressings or sauces.

You may have to grill your server a little to get the information you need. (I have a friend who always tells the server she's diabetic to make sure he *really* checks for sugar.) If you ask for the oil and vinegar cruets to dress your salad, you're guaranteed the dressing is sugar free.

The Level One Carbos meal is a little more restrictive when you're eating out. It must be fat-free so that all those carbohydrates are burned off rather than stored as fat. When eating a Carbo meal:

- Watch out for sugars and hidden Funky Foods.
- Avoid anything from the Proteins/Fats group; meat and cheese on that sandwich would throw your system into a tizzy.

Here are samples of perfect Somersize

meals at almost any type of restaurant you might encounter:

Italian: Here's a menu from my favorite restaurant, Coco Pazzo, in New York City. I'd first decide if I wanted a Proteins/Fats meal or a Carbos meal. If I wanted the protein, I'd first choose a protein entrée. The fish with herbs and lemon is a good choice or the chicken stuffed with onion. But almost all the entrées are fine—I'd just say no to any potatoes or to the cranberry beans that accompany the tuna. Then I'd choose an appetizer—probably the portobello mushrooms, but any of these appetizers will go with a Proteins/Fats meal. I'd be wary of the calamari, though, which may be battered in white flour—both a Funky Food and a Proteins/Fats and Carbos combination. I'd also order a salad: any of these three, but probably the baby artichoke salad with Parmesan.

Coco Pazzo Dinner Menu

Gli Antipasti

Vegetali alla Griglia
Assortment of grilled vegetables topped with a tarragon dressing

Calamari Fritti con Zucchini
Squid cut into rings and lightly fried with zucchini and parsley

Filetto di Tonno al Pepe Nero
Seared tuna rolled in black pepper, served on a bed of organic mixed greens

Antipasti Misto
Assorted marinated vegetables, salami, and cheeses from Tuscany

Insalata di Fagiolini e Pecorino con Olio Tartufo
Salad of French green beans and julienne of pecorino cheese dressed with white truffle oil

Portobello alla Griglia al Profumo del Rosmarino
Portobello mushroom caps grilled with rosemary

Pesce in Carpione
Sweet and sour Italian-style sardines served on a bed of baby spinach

Minestra del Giorno
Homemade soup, changes daily

Le Paste

Tagliatelle Angiolina
Homemade pasta tossed with blended fresh

tomatoes, Parmesan cheese, basil, and extra-virgin olive oil

Maccheroncini al Pepolino
Rectangles of fresh egg pasta with a rich tomato sauce flavored with fresh thyme and grated aged pecorino

Spaghetti del Norcino
. . . with crumbled hot and sweet sausage and tomato sauce

Fettuccine con Tartufo Nero e Funghi
Homemade flat noodles tossed with fresh aspara-gus, shavings of black truffles, and sautéed oyster mushrooms

Spaghetti con Vongole
. . . with a sauté of manila clams in the shell

Trofie al Pesto
Homemade semolina trofie with pesto, string beans, and potatoes

Risotto del Giorno
Carnaroli rice, ingredients change daily

Smaller portions of pasta are available as appetizers

I Secondi

Pesce Arrosto del Giorno
Whole fish of the day roasted with fresh herbs and lemon

Rollatina di Salmone
Salmon fillets rolled with basil, sautéed with sesame seeds, and served on a bed of baby cabbage

Pescatrice al Forno con Lenticchie
Baked monkfish served on a bed of lentil salad, finished with a basil dressing

Cernia al Tegame
Pan-sautéed grouper dressed with an onion and leek confit

Tonno alla Griglia con Fagioli all'Uccelletto
Grilled tuna with cranberry beans and sautéed dandelion greens

Filetto di Branzino in Brodetto
Fillet of bass stewed in a light mint broth with fresh tomatoes, topped with crispy onions

Bistecca Fiorentina
Rib-eye steak grilled on the bone, Florentine style

Fegato al Burro Nero e Salvia
Thinly sliced calf's liver sautéed with butter and fresh sage, topped with watercress

Polleto Farcito di Cipolla
Organic baby chicken stuffed with caramelized onions in a balsamic vinegar sauce

Battuta di Pollo
Lemon marinated chicken paillard served with arugula and tomato

Agnello con Peperonata
Grilled rack of lamb served with a vegetable "peperonata" and a galette of potatoes

Costoletta alla Milanese
Thinly pounded veal chop on the bone, breaded with herbs and served with a salad of mizuna, cherry tomatoes, and red onion

Le Nostre Patatine
Tuscan fried potatoes and herbs

Le Insalate

Insalata ai Sette Vegetali
Chopped vegetables and baby lettuces with vinaigrette

Insalata di Stagione
Seasonal green salad

Insalata di Carciofini
Thin shavings of raw baby artichokes and Parme-san cheese dressed with fresh lemon and extra virgin olive oil

Executive Chef: Maurizio Marfoglia

Now, if I wanted a Carbo meal, things would be a little more challenging. I'd have pasta—the *Fettuccine con Tartufo Nero e Funghi* is the only dish that doesn't seem to be combined with a Proteins/Fats. I'd double check to make sure the pasta was made with whole wheat rather than white flour (usually you can request whole wheat pasta or bring your own as long as you are willing to pay full price). I'd also order a Veggie appetizer like the Portobello mushroom caps or the grilled vegetables. I'd make sure there was no fat in the dressing or preparation. I could have a salad only if there was no fat in the dressing and they left off the Parmesan cheese. That is a lot of special requests! The kitchen would probably hate you. You can see how much more exciting the Protein/Fat meal would be. I would attempt to eat this Carbo meal only on Level Two, so I could have oil and a little cheese.

Mexican: Mexican cuisine tends to include a lot of cornmeal or flour tortillas with meat, poultry, cheese, and fish. But Mexican menus always offer chicken fajitas with grilled onions and peppers, which I eat with a lot of salsa for flavor, but without the flour tortilla. A taco salad—without the tortilla shell, beans, or guacamole—is another good option.

Japanese: Sashimi or sushi and vegetables are perfect for a Protein/Fat meal—just don't eat the sushi rice. Soba noodles are one of the few Carbos meals you can order in a restaurant—buckwheat noodles and vegetables with no fat. Sometimes a hard-boiled egg will accompany the dish—don't eat it.

French: People think French restaurants are *forbidden* when you're trying to lose weight, but they're perfect for Somersizing. The French rarely ever eat potatoes, rice, noodles, or any other type of carbohydrate with meat, fish, or chicken. Enjoy any of these dishes with a beautiful sauce and plenty of fresh vegetables. And don't forget the cheese plate for dessert.

Chinese: I find Chinese food the most difficult to Somersize. The sauces are loaded with cornstarch and sugar, and even the soups often contain wontons (Carbos) stuffed with ground meat (Proteins/Fats). But I can safely order steamed vegetables with brown rice, and I season them with soy sauce, which contains a trace amount of protein that won't affect the digestive system.

American: American or Continental restaurants always offer some form of meat and potatoes. It's easiest to just avoid the potatoes and any other carbohydrate. Order the meat, chicken, or fish with vegetables and a salad with dressing of your choice. Eat a burger (turkey or ground beef) without the bun. If you're lucky enough to stumble on a pizzeria that offers a whole wheat crust (such as the Continental Hotel at Disney World), grab it. Just don't have it with cheese. If the pizza is brushed with a little olive oil, you'll have to save it for Level Two.

4. What happens if I skip a meal?
Don't do it! Whether you're eating at home or dining in restaurants, make sure not to skip meals. Your mother always told you that breakfast is the most important meal of the day, right? In many ways, she was correct. Your body has been fasting

while you sleep, so when you wake up in the morning, you have gone for some eight to ten hours without food. If you skip breakfast and don't eat until lunch, your body has gone for twelve to fourteen hours without food. When you finally eat lunch, your body's survival instinct kicks in. It doesn't know when you're going to feed it again, so it hangs on to every morsel instead of properly processing the food. Remember to eat at least three meals a day —or as many as six mini-meals throughout the day, if you prefer.

5. *Can I Somersize part of the time and eat as I'm used to the rest of the time?*

As long as you are following *all* the Level One guidelines, you can eat until you are satisfied and comfortably full and still lose weight. But you cannot Somersize half-heartedly in the beginning. Your body is being retrained to burn your fat reserves. Don't confuse it by slipping up with bad combinations or Funky Foods. Besides, you have so many choices that there is no need to slip up. You will love eating this way and seeing the amazing results.

Some people see results immediately and lose five to ten pounds in the first week. Others don't see results until the second, third, or even fourth week. Be patient, and be diligent! Your body is detoxifying from all the sugar and chemicals and bad combinations it has become accustomed to. You *will* see results.

6. *I'm a vegetarian. What are my options on the Somersize program?*

It's a little tougher to eat vegetarian on the program because so many of the easiest meals include a protein like chicken or fish. But you can make wonderful Carbos meals out of whole wheat pasta or brown or wild rice and vegetables. You can also cook with rice and beans—good protein sources, although we include them in the carbo group—or add tofu to fresh vegetables. Use textured vegetable protein to make burgers; add it to chilis, soys, and sauces. Look in the second half of this book for a host of meatless appetizers and main dishes. Vegans can have rice milk (not soy milk) on their carbo breakfast cereal.

7. *I like to put milk in my coffee. Is that okay?*

As you know, whole milk and low-fat milk are Funky Foods and are not allowed on the Level One program. The only kind of milk you can have is nonfat (skim) milk, which is categorized as a carbohydrate because it has no fat. Therefore, you may have nonfat milk in your decaf coffee when you are having a

> You are Somersizing to look
>
> and feel your very best so you
>
> can enjoy all this beautiful
>
> world has to offer.

Carbos meal or a Carbos and Veggies meal. But when you are having a Proteins/Fats meal or a Proteins/Fats and Veggies meal, you cannot use any milk in your decaf coffee because milk has carbohydrates that we do not mix with proteins. I know it may sound strange, but you should use cream in your coffee when you are having proteins because cream can be digested more easily with proteins. Vegans can use rice milk in their coffee with a Carbos meal, or soy milk in their coffee with a Proteins/Fats meal.

8. *I love eating pasta, but I'm having a hard time eating it on Level One with no fat. Any suggestions?*

On Level One, you have to make some adjustments when you eat pasta, but you don't have to eliminate it altogether. First, you must find whole-grain pasta and then top it with a sauce that contains no oil, butter, or cheese. You probably will have a difficult time eating Level One pasta meals in restaurants, but it is possible to make your own sauce with no added fat. (See my Level One Simple Tomato, Basil, and Garlic Sauce, page 145.) When you make your nonfat sauce, start by sautéing your onions and garlic in a little tomato juice rather than in olive oil. Then add fresh or canned tomatoes and any of your favorite steamed or grilled vegetables with plenty of fresh herbs. Sorry, no cheese! Finally, try whole-grain pasta with fresh vegetables and soy sauce. It's delicious.

9. *I crave desserts. What can I eat on Level One to satisfy my sweet tooth?*

If you are used to eating a lot of sugar, you may go through a period of withdrawal when you begin Level One. Fruit is a natural form of sugar that will help satisfy your cravings. Look for fruit sorbets or fruit popsicles sweetened only with fruit juice. Just make sure you wait two hours after your last meal before you have any fruit. Also, take a look at my recipes for Sugarless Cheesecake (page 186) and Decaf Coffee Granita (page 187).

10. *What do I do when I am having dinner at someone's house?*

I'm sure you will be so excited about your new lifestyle that you will love sharing it with your hosts and other dinner guests. However, if you do not care to advertise your new way of eating at a dinner party, you can usually disguise your eating habits without offending your hosts. Put the passed bread on your plate and break it into two pieces. No one will notice that you haven't eaten any. Your salad course is almost always Somersized; just eat around the carrots. Usually, dinner is some type of meat or fish served with rice, pasta, potatoes, or vegetables. Eat the entrée with the exception of carbohydrates and you will have no problem.

The most difficult situation occurs when you are served some type of casserole or pasta made with white flour and bad combinations. Just eat a small portion and get right back on Level One the following day. As far as dessert, most hosts will understand if you pass. But if you must have a little so as not to offend, have a taste and pour on the compliments!

For your first few days or weeks on the program, you might want to make a copy of this page and slip it into your purse or wallet. Somersizing will soon become second nature to you, but this summary will help remind you of the plan until you no longer need it for reference.

1. Eliminate all Funky Foods.
2. Eat Fruits alone, on an empty stomach.
3. Eat Proteins/Fats with Veggies.
4. Eat Carbos with Veggies and no fat.
5. Keep Proteins/Fats separate from Carbos.
6. Wait three hours between meals if switching from a Proteins/Fats meal to a Carbos meal, or vice versa.
7. Do not skip meals. Eat three meals a day, and eat until you feel satisfied and comfortably full.

PROTEINS AND FATS

Butter	Mayonnaise
Cheese	Meat
Cream	Oil
Eggs	Poultry
Fish	Sour cream

VEGGIES

Asparagus	Green beans
Broccoli	Lettuce
Cauliflower	Mushrooms
Celery	Spinach
Cucumber	Tomato
Eggplant	Zucchini

CARBOS

Beans	Whole-grain breads,
Mustard	cereals, pastas
Nonfat milk products	

FRUITS

Apples	Oranges
Berries	Papaya
Grapes	Peaches
Mangoes	Pears
Melons	Plums
Nectarines	

Eliminate Funky Foods

SUGARS

Beets	Maple syrup
Carrots	Molasses
Corn syrup	Sugar
Honey	

STARCHES

Bananas	Potatoes
Corn	Sweet potatoes
Pasta made from semolina or white flour	White flour
	White rice
	Winter squashes
Popcorn	

COMBO PROTEINS/FATS AND CARBOS

Avocados	Nuts
Coconuts	Olives
Liver	Tofu
Low-fat or whole milk	

CAFFEINE AND ALCOHOL

Alcoholic beverages
Caffeinated coffees, teas, and sodas
Cocoa

CHAPTER EIGHT

It's Up to You

UNDERSTANDING YOUR PATTERNS OF BEHAVIOR

More than twenty years ago, when I started to realize I had to make a change in my eating habits, it was important for me to approach it in the same way that I have approached all the problems in my life: go back and look honestly at my patterns of behavior. I was at a point where I was either going to be fighting fat for the rest of my life or I had to make some major changes. I saw other women my age starting to become the pear shape of so many older women and I decided that was undesirable and unnecessary.

Why was I on a diet merry-go-round? How could I get control of my weight, rather than my weight being in control of me? I had to look at my patterns and see the things I was doing to myself that were destructive: eating when I was upset, tired,

happy—all the time! When I found a pattern in my actions that I was able to recognize and understand, I made the decision to change. I realized it was up to me.

So many people who have experienced miraculous results on the Somersize program started it because they were desperate. They were unhappy with their bodies and unhappy with themselves. They had tried many diets, but were unable to see that what they really needed to do was change their attitudes toward eating and toward food. They had to break with the idea of food as good and bad—which only leads to deprivation and bingeing. They had to accept food in proper combinations as a pleasurable, nourishing part of life. These people were unhappy, but they came to realize that this unhappiness was within their power to change.

In essence, the theory behind Somersizing is to find an easy, livable way to look and feel your best, enjoy life, eat great food, and have a healthy body that you're happy with and a digestive system and metabolism that work at an optimum level.

Here's what happened with me. All my life I've tried to be perfect. I know there are a lot of you reading this book who can identify with me. I always wondered why perfection was so important. Why do I jump out of a nice, comfortable chair if I notice a painting on the wall is a little crooked? Why do I make my own pastry crust when frozen will do almost as well? Because I want everything to be perfect! I realize now that my perfectionism relates back to my childhood. If only I could have been a perfect daughter, maybe my dad wouldn't have drunk so much. As a child, I thought I could control an out-of-control environment by being the best, the smartest, the funniest, the most talented. I wanted to *please*! If I could only do that, then peace would come to our crazy household.

All these years and hundreds of hours of

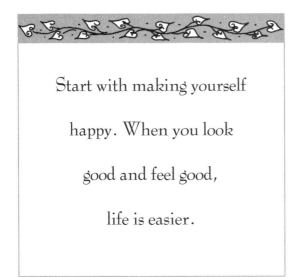

Start with making yourself happy. When you look good and feel good, life is easier.

therapy later, I have realized that there was no way I could have changed the situation of my childhood, no matter how perfectly I behaved. But the pattern of behavior had already been set in place. As a result, I am now a woman who tries very hard to do everything well. Sometimes I find myself exhausted and feeling used or unappreciated. That's when I realize I am having an emotional slip.

There is a big emotional price to pay for trying to have it all. I try to be a perfect wife, perfect mother, and perfect grandmother while giving my best to my career. I must also run the house, do the shopping, cook interesting meals, decorate, inspire my mind, and keep this fifty-year-old body in tiptop, toned shape. I have had to find a way to do all this that makes life worth living.

That's why Somersizing has been such a huge relief for me. It allows me to relax, enjoy meals, and have good conversations without guilt and deprivation. When I remember how much time I used to spend thinking about food, and what to eat and what not to eat and worrying about how I looked and felt, I truly regret all the minutes and hours I could have been doing something more pleasurable and worthwhile.

Somersizing is like a little secret. Once you understand it, it becomes so easy—just another part of your life. I no longer think about what is a carbohydrate and what is a protein. I've been doing it for so long, I just *know* it. I remember when I was in therapy; nothing made any sense at first. I felt confused and agitated. Then one day it was as if a light bulb had gone on. Suddenly I saw my behaviors repeating themselves. I realized I had to change my behavior patterns if I were to grow and move forward.

This is what I'm trying to teach you in Somersizing. You've tried the diets over and over. You keep going back to your old patterns of eating—and the same old body returns (and then some). Remember, this is something you're doing for yourself. You're not trying to look attractive for someone else; you're Somersizing to look and feel your very best so you can enjoy all this beautiful world has to offer. No one will be as sorry as you if you don't get what you want out of life.

Somersizing is a shift in your thinking. It's not a short-term diet. In fact, if you are approaching it this way, I suggest that you not do it at all. It is important to embrace Somersizing as something you can do for the rest of your life. I know *I* will. I plan to be thin and in control of my weight for the rest of my life. Somersizing offers me this gift. It's there for you, too, but *you* must decide to change your eating patterns.

BE FIT, NOT FANATIC!

I exercise enough to keep toned, but not Jane Fonda–perfect. Because I don't spend hours at the gym, I *do* have time to read those books on my night table (sometimes while using my ThighMaster!). I ride my bike with Alan, I hike with my family, I take vacations. I now know I can eat anywhere my family does—even those pile-your-plate restaurants at the beach—and not sacrifice my physical well-being.

Exercise is an important part of any weight-loss program. That doesn't mean you have to spend three hours a day taking aerobics classes. Just get yourself out and start moving. My motto is, "Be fit, not fanatic." Take a walk—just a twenty-minute walk—in the morning or the afternoon. Play tag with your kids. Choose the stairs instead of the elevator. Take an active look at your activity level. Exercise helps you build lean muscle mass, which is a key element in losing weight. Lean muscle mass helps you burn fat twenty-four hours a day! Find an activity that brings you enjoyment —it doesn't have to cost money, it just has to get you moving.

Here's how I make movement a part of my daily life. I never go the gym. I've never *been* to a gym! I do what my body tells me it needs to do for me to look and feel my best—and I get that message by standing in front of a mirror and looking at myself without sucking in my stomach or flexing my muscles.

Physically, I'm a lazy, lazy person. So three times a week, my son-in-law, Frank Buffa, comes over and takes me through a routine of mat work and isometric exercises that include situps, calf raises (yes, even our calves sag as we get older), and stretching, to increase flexibility.

I really do this. I keep my ThighMaster and my ButtMaster on the floor right by my bed, so I trip over them when I get up and can't possibly forget to use them.

The rest of the activity in my life is really a form of pleasure. I ride my bike on the beach in Los Angeles. It's a wonderful way to get fresh air, look at the interesting people on the boardwalk, and talk to Alan (we have

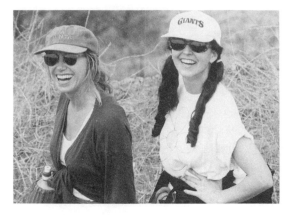

My daughter-in-law, Caroline, and me in the Malibu mountains. Exercising is a family affair.

a tandem bike). We hike all over the Malibu mountains as a family, sometimes for two hours, sometimes for eight hours. We take along a picnic and make a real pleasure trip out of it. It's a great way to connect with my family, and it's a good workout for my body. If we're on a winter vacation, we cross-country ski. And in the summer, I love getting in and out of the swimming pool all day. I also love to do Tai Chi exercises when I am working at the studio because it takes no space. You can find these in my video *Think Great, Look Great* (CBS/Fox Videos).

I'm not a rigid or scheduled person. Movement is an organic part of my life. Rather than saying, "Oh, I have to go to the gym for an hour today," I take a long walk on the beach. Movement is as simple as choosing to play in the pool with your kids instead of sitting by the side. I've learned over the years to listen to my inner voice, which tells me "I'm hungry" or "I need to get some fresh air" or "I need to sleep." Once you trust yourself, you'll find balance.

The answers are within us. We must train ourselves to listen for them.

In a short while, Somersizing will be as second nature to you as it is to me. I no longer have to be perfect. As human beings, we are imperfect. After you have lost all the weight you desire, you will graduate to maintenance—a phase which allows you to be your own best judge of your eating. When I eat a meal that is not perfectly Somersized, I don't beat myself up. I just realize that I've created an imbalance, and I go back to Level One until my body feels right again.

I don't live with a bunch of "nevers"— *never* have fat, *never* have dessert, *never* have wine, *never* have fun. When we impose rigid rules on ourselves, eventually we will fail because we are not perfect. This is an opportunity for you to enjoy your imperfections. Live life, eat great, be happy, love yourself.

It starts with making yourself happy. When we look good and feel good, life is easier.

CHAPTER NINE

Level Two: A Lifestyle You Can Live With

Congratulations! You've made it to your goal weight! Wasn't it easy? Isn't Somersizing the most pleasurable way to lose weight that you've ever tried? I'm sure you look great with your new figure in those shapely clothes you thought you'd never fit into again. I bet you've been answering a lot of questions about how you lost the weight, right? Your friends, family, and coworkers are probably hounding you for information so they can follow your lead.

Now it's time to graduate to Level Two, where you'll learn how to Somersize for the rest of your life. Level Two is really an extension of Level One, with a few indulgences here and there. Or, if your goal is to stabilize your digestion without losing excess body weight, you may enter the Somersize eating plan at Level Two.

By eliminating Funky Foods on Level One, you've stabilized your blood sugar levels. You're avoiding sugar highs and lows.

Rather than going from quick energy fix to quick energy fix of refined carbohydrates, you have trained your body to use your fat reserves as an energy source. You have conditioned your system to digest quickly and efficiently by cutting out bad food combinations.

So now your body is in great shape and can handle a few imbalances. But you are the only one who can determine how much imbalance you can handle. Some people have to stay very close to the Level One guidelines, with a minor imbalance here and there, in order to maintain their weight. Other people find they can take in quite a few imbalances and still maintain their weight. By using trial and error, you'll soon know what your body can handle.

There are specific guidelines necessary to lose weight in Level One, and if you've gotten down to your goal weight, you have followed them diligently. I wish I could give you specific guidelines for Level Two, but that's the beauty of it: there are *no* hard and fast rules. You are in control of your body, and you need to find a rhythm you can live with for the rest of your life.

The great thing is that by experimenting with imbalances, you can always find your equilibrium. Moderation is the key to maintaining your weight. I find that if I eat a Level One lunch, like a grilled chicken salad with warm goat cheese, julienned vegetables, and balsamic vinaigrette, every now and then I can add a piece of flourless chocolate cake for dessert without upsetting my system too much. But if I ate a piece of flourless chocolate cake *every day* with an otherwise Level One lunch, it would catch up with me. And if I ate the grilled chicken salad along with a white-bread roll *and* the cake, I'd be living in Bloat City.

MIXING PROTEINS/FATS AND CARBOS

For me, the combination of Proteins/Fats and Carbos is tough on my body, so even on Level Two I try to keep them completely separate. Do I always succeed? No, of course not. Sometimes I just *have* to have turkey with mashed potatoes and gravy. So I have it. And then I eat Level One meals for a good while, until my system gets back in balance.

That's how Level Two works; you eat mostly on Level One and decide when you want to treat yourself. Sometimes I stay close to Level One with frequent but small little treats here and there, like a little olive oil on my pasta or some wild rice in my chicken soup. I stay strictly on Level One for a series of meals and then have a big treat, like a piece of birthday cake with buttercream frosting or a wild mushroom risotto with Parmesan cheese. And a couple times a year I *really* treat myself and eat french fries!

Last time Alan and I were in New York, we were doing the *Regis and Kathie Lee Show* and we ran into Cheryl Ladd. I told her we were going to one of our favorite restaurants for lunch, Coco Pazzo. She had been there the night before and had what she said were the most incredible french fries of her life.

She was right. These fries were *to die for:* hot, crispy, perfectly salted. And they were served with fried herbs, so with every few bites you would get a mouthful of fried tarragon or fried sage—unbelievable! I had a plate of fries, a green salad, and a glass of red wine. An exquisite lunch, and worth every

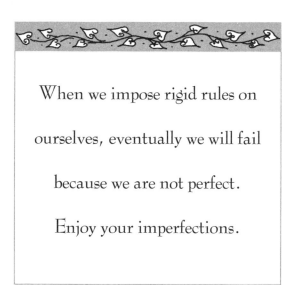

When we impose rigid rules on ourselves, eventually we will fail because we are not perfect.

Enjoy your imperfections.

bite. It was no problem living on Level One for a while to get back my balance.

Generally I find that on Level Two I can add a little bit of fat in my Carbos meals without causing a problem. I often have whole-grain pasta or brown rice for lunch with vegetables. On Level One I have no oil with this meal, but on Level Two I can sauté the veggies in some oil and have a more flavorful stir-fry without causing a significant imbalance.

But I find that I bloat if I add any kind of meat to my pasta or brown rice. The protein in combination with the Carbos is harder on my body than fat in combination with the Carbos. Wild rice is an exception for me; I find that it's easier on my system than other Carbos, and I don't seem to have a problem eating it with Proteins/Fats on Level Two.

If I'm going to have a sandwich, I usually still have a vegetarian sandwich on whole-grain bread, but every now and then I add some avocado. The avocado has fat in it, but as long as I don't add meat as well, I generally find I do not have a problem. I also might add a little mayonnaise or olive oil, depending on the sandwich. And if I feel like having a meat or tuna sandwich, then I usually stick to Level One and use lettuce cups instead of bread. (If I were to eat bread with meat or tuna, it would definitely be whole-grain bread.)

MIXING FRUIT

I still try to eat the Fruits group completely separately. The only fruit I play around with is berries, because berries are easier for me to digest than other fruits. They have a very high fiber content and give me very little

A piping hot frittata and a crispy apple tart—delicious even from my old stove (before I remodeled my kitchen).

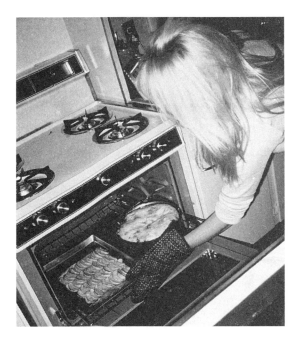

trouble when I combine them with other foods in moderation. When I get tired of toast with nonfat cottage cheese or nonfat yogurt, I use a little berry jam (sweetened with fruit juice, not sugar—like Polaner All Fruit) on my toast in the morning. Or sometimes I top whole wheat pancakes with homemade raspberry sauce (raspberries, lemon, and a little sweetener). Regular pancakes with butter and maple syrup would create a huge imbalance, whereas whole wheat or buckwheat pancakes with raspberry sauce cause less of an imbalance and still satisfy my craving.

I also like to use berries in tarts and pies made with whole wheat crusts. It's certainly not Level One fare, but it is easier on your system than an apple tart or a pumpkin pie. For breakfast or a snack in the afternoon, I like to have fresh berries with nonfat yogurt. And I may also add a few products that are sweetened with fruit juice. At natural foods stores you can find cereals made from spelt, amaranth, and kamut flakes that are sweetened with a little fruit juice. They provide a nice change in the morning.

ADDING SOME SUGAR AND FUNKY FOODS

As far as sugar goes, I loosen the reins a little. I'm not quite as diligent about hunting for sugar in sauces and salad dressings. If I'm at a restaurant, I don't worry about eating a prepared blue cheese dressing on my salad, even if it has a little sugar in it. It's not enough to cause a problem for me in Level Two as long as I'm not having any Carbos. I continue to

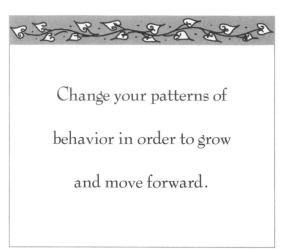

Change your patterns of behavior in order to grow and move forward.

avoid gravy made with white flour and very sweet sauces, like barbecue sauce. And I watch out for those thick Chinese sauces made with sugar and cornstarch. Most restaurants are happy to prepare your food without these ingredients.

And how about desserts? Every now and then it's okay to enjoy a dessert. On Level Two I probably eat dessert once a week; however, you may be able to eat more or less depending on your system and whether or not you have any health problems. Some desserts are more appropriate for Somersize Level Two than others. I still stay away from the extremely sugary ones.

Take a look at the sugar content in pecan pie, for example. The filling alone is made from ½ cup of corn syrup and 1 cup of brown sugar! Add the nuts, which are a Funky Food, the butter, which is a Proteins/Fats, and the crust, which is made from butter and white flour, and you have a poorly combined Proteins/Fats–Carbos–Funky Food concoction sure to send your system into a tizzy. My recipe for berry pie uses only

⅓ cup of sugar in the filling—a much better option for Somersizing purposes.

But the beauty of this program is that if you really want it, you can have the pecan pie—you just have to eat back on Level One for a longer period.

Another good dessert option after a Proteins/Fats meal is a piece of cheesecake with fresh berries. Cheesecake is often lower in sugar than other desserts (especially my Sugarless Cheesecake, page 186) and is made mostly of eggs, cream cheese, sour cream, lemon juice, and sometimes a touch of flour or cornstarch. Pudding, crème brûlée, chocolate mousse, and even ice cream are generally lower in sugar than most other desserts and do not have white flour, as do many pastries. Flourless chocolate cake is a great Level Two option, or strawberries dipped in chocolate with freshly whipped cream!

I can really eat these desserts and maintain my weight if I am Somersizing properly.

Check out my recipes for Level Two desserts. You'll be knocked out by how great they are. They are all relatively low in sugar, and I use whole wheat pastry flour instead of all-purpose white flour. I tried experimenting with nonfat desserts or desserts made with artificial sweeteners and they didn't taste great. It was always a qualified "good." Then my son-in-law, Frank, my personal trainer, said to me, "You should not make diet desserts. Desserts are not diet food. Eat real desserts, but not too often." He's absolutely right. (I do make an exception for my sugarless Level One cheesecake.)

YOU'RE THE BOSS

As far as Level Two goes, you are the boss. Maybe you don't miss sweets as much as you miss white bread. Then save your treats for a great baguette or a chewy sourdough roll. Or if it's standard pasta you're craving, eat mostly Level One meals and then indulge yourself with a little pasta fix. It's up to you. I bring whole wheat pasta to my favorite Italian restaurant and ask the kitchen to use it instead of the usual white pasta. They never seem to mind, as long as I pay full price for my dish. I still stay away from meat sauce with my whole-grain pasta because the combination makes me bloat.

The last time I ate Italian food, I started with an arugula and radicchio salad with

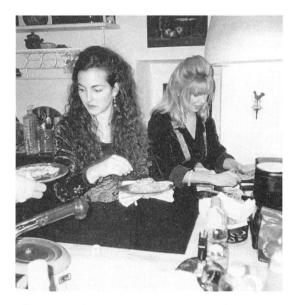

Serving Christmas dinner with my daughter-in-law, Caroline.

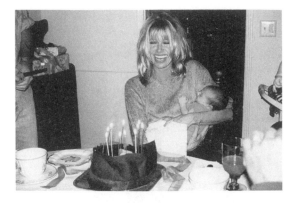

My forty-ninth birthday, with the incredible Decadent Chocolate Cake (page 200) and my new granddaughter.

shaved Parmesan cheese and an olive oil, lemon, and garlic dressing. Then I had whole wheat pasta with a wild mushroom and tomato sauce and a glass of red wine. This is predominantly a Carbos and Veggies meal, but I did have some Proteins/Fats (some oil in the salad dressing and the pasta sauce and Parmesan cheese on the salad and the pasta). After this meal I did not order a dessert because I felt I had used up my imbalances with the addition of the oil, cheese, and wine.

But let's say I had the salad with roasted chicken and grilled vegetables. In that case, I might have enjoyed my glass of red wine *and* a dessert. Also remember, on Level Two you can take caffeine and sugary colas (if you have to have them) as optional imbalances.

How you choose your imbalances depends on many factors. How many imbalances have you had today and how big were they? Did you have a dessert or did you have a potato? How many big imbalances have you had this week?

Don't get cocky with your new figure! The pounds can creep right back on if you're not careful. If you notice that you're gaining a couple pounds, or if you feel sluggish, go back to Level One until you get rid of the problem. Stay on top of the new you. Take care of your body.

Also, control your portion size. On Level One you can eat until you are satisfied and comfortable, as long as you follow *all* the Level One guidelines. In fact, you'll find that you don't want to overeat. But on Level Two, you must consider limiting your portions. You can't have it both ways. I find that the bonus of Level One is that I can eat as much as I want. The bonus of Level Two is that you have more variety, but you must limit your portions moderately.

WINE AND CHOCOLATE

Recent studies have shown that red wine can have beneficial effects on the heart by helping keep your arteries clear. How wonderful! I have incorporated it in moderation on Level Two. A glass or two every now and then with your meals is perfectly fine. I also use wine in many of my Level Two recipes. It creates only a slight imbalance because most of the alcohol is cooked off in the heating process. In fact, I sometimes cook with wine even on Level One because it wonderfully enhances the flavor of my meals and does not seem to disrupt my system.

Now for chocolate. Oh yes, the decadent, delicious treat I can't seem to live without. And I don't have to! Dark chocolate (made from at least 60 percent cocoa) is relatively low in sugar and does not create a huge imbalance for me. I love to eat a square every once in a while in the afternoon between meals. I also make what taste like sinful desserts from dark chocolate on occasion.

A SAMPLE WEEK

From week to week, my meal plans vary greatly on Level Two. As with Level One, I want to share one particular week of meals with you because it is a good model in terms of balancing Proteins/Fats and Carbos and getting plenty of Fruits and Veggies. You will see a combination of Level One meals and Level Two meals. Remember, your body may be able to handle different levels of imbalances depending on your particular metabolism. This sample week reflects how many imbalances I can handle and still maintain my weight. To help you see how I choose my treats, I have put an asterisk next to the items that are Level Two.

SUNDAY
9:00 Breakfast—Proteins/Fats and Veggies
    Zucchini Frittata (page 139)
    Decaf coffee

1:00 Lunch—Proteins/Fats and Veggies
    Turkey Sausage with Peppers and
        Onions (page 169)
    Green Salad with Artichoke Hearts and
        Red Wine Vinaigrette (page 107)
3:00 Snack—Fruits
    Fruit juice popsicle
7:00 Dinner—Carbos and Veggies
    Whole Wheat Pasta with Pine Nuts★
        (page 192)
    Steamed broccoli and cauliflower
        tossed in olive oil, salt, and pepper
    Green salad with Garlic Vinaigrette
        (page 95)
    Glass of red wine
    Rosemary tea
    (★I combined oil, a Protein/Fat, with a Carbos
    and Veggies meal, plus wine.)

MONDAY
9:00 Breakfast—Fruit
    Mango
9:30—Carbos
    Rye bagel with canola margarine★
    Decaf coffee
    (★I combined margarine, a Protein/Fat, with
    my Carbos breakfast.)

1:30 Lunch—Proteins/Fats and Veggies
    Grilled Chicken Salad with Sun-Dried
        Tomatoes and Goat Cheese
        (page 115)
    Decadent Chocolate Cake★ (page 200)
    (★This Level Two dessert has a little flour, sugar,
    and chocolate.)

7:30 Dinner—Proteins/Fats and Veggies
    Clay Pot Chicken and Leeks (page 159)
    Celery Root Puree (page 98)
    Butter lettuce salad with Garlic Vinai-
        grette (page 95)

7:30 *Breakfast—Fruits*
    Cantaloupe
    Decaf coffee

12:00 *Lunch—Carbos and Veggies*
    Stir-Fried Vegetables (page 100), with
      brown rice★
    (★I added oil, a Protein/Fat, to a Carbos and
    Veggies meal.)

3:00 *Snack—Funky Food*
    A square or two of dark chocolate★
    (★Lower in sugar than most chocolates, it still
    creates the least imbalance when eaten alone.)

7:00 *Dinner—Proteins/Fats and Veggies*
    Stuffed Zucchini (page 102)
    Medallions of Lamb (page 178)
    Green salad with dressing of
      your choice
    Glass of red wine★
    (★wine)

WEDNESDAY

7:30 *Breakfast—Proteins/Fats and Veggies*
    Egg white omelet with sausage
      and cheese
    Decaf coffee

1:00 *Lunch—Carbos and Veggies*
    Lentil Soup (page 130)
    Whole-grain crackers
    Mixed green salad with Italian
      dressing★
    (★I added a little oil, a Protein/Fat, to a
    Carbos and Veggies meal.)

4:00 *Snack—Carbos*
    Nonfat yogurt with berries★
    (★I mixed Carbos with Fruits.)

7:30 *Dinner—Proteins/Fats and Veggies*
    Turkey Meatloaf (page 168)
    Celery Root Puree (page 98)
    Green Beans with Garlic Vinaigrette
      (page 95)

THURSDAY

7:30 *Breakfast—Carbos and Veggies*
    Whole wheat toast with sliced tomato
      and basil

10:00 *Snack—Fruits*
    Orange

12:30 *Lunch—Carbos and Veggies*
    Whole-grain pasta with Basil Pesto★
      (page 79)
    Green salad with romaine, red cabbage,
      celery, and Red Wine Vinaigrette
      (page 107)
    Glass of red wine
    (★I combined oil and cheese, Proteins/Fats,
    with my Carbos and Veggies, plus wine.)

6:30 *Dinner—Proteins/Fats and Veggies*
    Chicken Paillard with Lemon-Parsley
      Butter and Seared Red Chard
      (page 160)
    Steamed asparagus
    Frozen Chocolate Mousse with
      whipped cream★ (page 198)
    (★This Level Two dessert has chocolate and
    a little sugar.)

FRIDAY

7:00 *Breakfast—Proteins/Fats and Veggies*
    Scrambled eggs with onion, salsa,
      and cilantro
    Decaf coffee

> Accept food in proper
>
> combinations as a pleasurable,
>
> nourishing part of life.

1:00 Lunch—Proteins/Fats and Veggies
Oriental Turkey Meatball Soup
(page 128)

3:30 Snack—Fruits
Raspberry sorbet (fruit juice
sweetened, no sugar)

7:30 Dinner—Proteins/Fats and Veggies
Citrus-Marinated Barbecued Shrimp
with Fresh Arugula (page 148)
Summer Squash Medley (page 91)
Green salad with Garlic Vinaigrette
(page 95)
Glass of white wine
Lemon Curd Tart★ (page 196)
(★This Level Two dessert has a little whole
wheat flour and honey, plus I had wine.)

S A T U R D A Y
8:00 Breakfast—Fruits
Fruit Smoothie (page 88)

8:30—Carbos
Whole-grain toast with berry jam★
(fruit juice sweetened, no sugar)
(★I mixed Carbos and Fruits.)

1:00 Lunch—Carbos and Veggies
Roasted Red Peppers and Grilled Bread
(page 81) with Pecorino cheese★
Baked Garlic (page 80)
Cannellini Bean Dip (page 74)
Tricoloré Salad with Balsamic
Vinaigrette★ (page 106)
(★I combined oil and cheese, Proteins/Fats,
with Carbos and Veggies.)

7:00 Dinner—Proteins/Fats and Veggies
Roasted Herbes de Provence Chicken
(page 164)
Green Beans with Garlic Vinaigrette
(page 95)
Baby Artichoke Salad (page 111)
Glass of red wine★
Fresh berries with whipped cream★
(★I combined Fruits with Proteins/Fats and
Veggies, plus a glass of wine.)

I have such a great time eating on Level
Two because I don't have to sacrifice anything. I certainly don't indulge myself every
time I have a craving, but I do it often
enough so that I never feel deprived.

You can continue to use all the Level
One recipes in Part Two of this book for
Level Two. In addition, I have included a
few recipes specific to Level Two. Good
luck in this new phase. You have such free-
dom; I just know you'll love it. Any questions you have will be answered by your
own body as you experiment with foods.

Eating this way is truly a pleasure. I'm
sure you will be the envy of all your
friends, who'll find it hard to believe what
wonderful foods you eat while keeping
your beautiful figure.

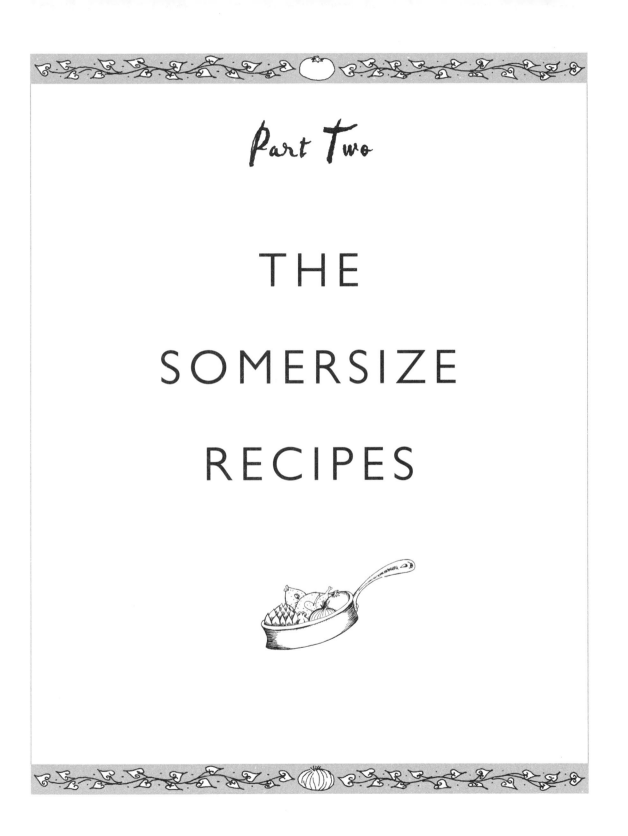

Part Two

THE

SOMERSIZE

RECIPES

CHAPTER TEN

❧

The Somersize Pantry

If you're used to using prepared foods when you cook and eat at home, you will need to make some adjustments. Most prepared foods include processed Funky Foods like sugar and white flour. But with a little preparation, you can learn to create fresh foods that taste much better and are far more nutritious.

I keep my refrigerator stocked with ingredients that allow me to prepare great meals in minutes. I like to shop at our local farmers' market on Saturdays and stock up for the week. Then on Sundays I do a little cooking: perhaps a pot of cannellini beans to make my delicious White Bean Garden Salad (page 191) or to throw into a fresh vegetable soup or puree as a dip for vegetables or a spread for sandwiches. Maybe I'll roast a chicken for a family dinner. The next day I'll use the leftover meat for a chicken salad, and then use the carcass to make my yummy Chicken Tomato Cilantro Soup (page 126) for the following night.

Having ingredients in the house makes coming home from work and preparing dinner so easy. The recipes in this book are fast and require minimal skill as a chef. As with any good recipe, the most important part is good-quality ingredients. Here are some of the ingredients I like to always have in my refrigerator and pantry. I can whip up Somersize meals in minutes when I have these supplies around.

Whole-Grain Pastas Whatever brand you choose, look for durum wheat, durum wheat semolina, or whole grains such as spelt or kamut in the list of ingredients. I also like whole wheat and artichoke or whole wheat and spinach pastas.

Rice Brown rice and wild rice. Make sure neither are blended with white rice of any sort.

Whole-Grain Bread Whole wheat,

pumpernickel (a form of rye), or rye bread—whatever kind you like. Keep an extra loaf in the freezer so you never run out. Check for hidden sugars, fats, fruits, or sweeteners. Choose totally natural breads made without honey, white flour, or fruit juice. And don't forget whole wheat pitas, whole wheat flat bread, and whole wheat tortillas; just make sure they're made without any fats.

Phyllo Dough Many types are whole wheat. Keep a box in the freezer for quick Level Two tarts and pastries.

Hot Cereals Oatmeal and Cream of Wheat.

Cold Cereals I like Shredded Wheat, Grape-Nuts, and Crispy Brown Rice. Again, check carefully on the labels for sugars and Funky Foods. Even All-Bran isn't "all bran"—it has added sugar.

Nonfat Cottage Cheese You can now get calcium-enriched cottage cheese. I recommend it.

Nonfat Yogurt Pavel's is my favorite brand, but it's sometimes hard to find.

Nonfat Milk Also called skim milk. Again, calcium-enriched is a plus.

Cheese Whatever kind you like. I usually keep Stilton or another good blue, Parmesan or Romano, goat, and feta cheeses on hand. Pecorino is another favorite of mine and sometimes I splurge on a triple cream like Camembert or Brie.

Butter Regular and unsalted.

Margarine If you're watching your cholesterol, canola oil margarine is a good alternative to butter. But I use margarine sparingly—if at all—because it's often loaded with chemicals and has little taste. Olive oil is another great butter substitute.

Fresh Eggs I get mine from the farmers' market for the freshest of fresh.

Mustard Yellow, whole-grain, and Dijon.

Mayonnaise Make sure it has no sugar added. Or make your own, with my easy recipe (see page 86).

Fresh Fish I always buy my fish the same day I eat it. My favorites are sea bass, trout, and tuna.

Meat I don't eat a lot of meat, but I like to keep a few things in the freezer to thaw for a quick meal. Pork chops, lean ground beef, steaks, and lamb chops.

Poultry I eat a lot of chicken. I have the butcher make a few packages with two chicken breasts in each. That way I can keep them in the freezer and thaw them quickly for an easy meal. I do the same with turkey cutlets—they're a nice alternative with a slightly different flavor. I also keep ground chicken and ground turkey on hand.

Beans—Dried, Canned, or Fresh I like cannellini beans, pinto beans, lentils, black-eyed peas, and garbanzo beans (also called chickpeas).

Oil I buy extra-virgin olive oil by the case. I use it in almost every meal. I also keep vegetable oils, like safflower or canola. And don't forget hot chili oil and roasted sesame oil to flavor those delicious Asian meals.

Vinegar Balsamic, red wine, and white wine vinegar are my household staples. Rice vinegar is good to have around for Asian dishes.

Lettuce I buy my lettuce on the weekend and wash, dry, and bag it so that I have easy salads all week long. You can also buy prewashed lettuce. I like red leaf, butter lettuce, romaine, radicchio, and endive.

Onions Brown, white, yellow, or red; also scallions and leeks.

Garlic And plenty of it. Sometimes I peel a few heads and keep the cloves in olive oil in the fridge for quick access.

Ginger For Asian recipes.

Soy Sauce For Asian recipes.

Fresh Veggies Whatever is in season and looks great—asparagus, broccoli, cauliflower, tomatoes, summer squash, zucchini, fennel, celery, celery root, green beans, bell peppers.

Fresh and Dried Herbs Basil, thyme, rosemary, parsley, tarragon, dill, mint, and cilantro are a few that I always like to have around.

Fresh Fruits I choose whatever is in season—apples, grapes, mangoes, papaya, melons, berries, and citrus fruits. Because their sugar content is so low, lemons and limes can be used to season foods from any of the four Somersize Food Groups.

Frozen Fruits Frozen fruits are great for Fruit Smoothies and Level Two pastries. I always have frozen berries and peaches on hand—and mangoes when I can find them.

Frozen Veggies I use frozen veggies only when I absolutely can't get them fresh. The flavor doesn't compare.

Canned Goods I always keep canned tomatoes on hand for easy-to-prepare sauces. I buy tomato sauce, crushed tomatoes, and whole peeled tomatoes. I also like hearts of palm, which are great in salads. Canned bamboo shoots are good for Asian dishes, and a few cans of tuna are nice to have around to throw into salads. I always

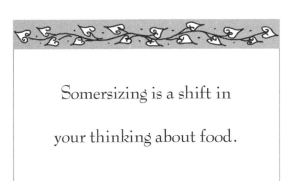

Somersizing is a shift in

your thinking about food.

keep cans of chicken and beef stock on hand for the times when I can't make my own.

COOKING TIPS

I don't like to waste food or time, so I love to cook big batches of foods ahead of time. Then I use them during the week for instant gourmet meals. For example, I'll prepare pesto when basil is in season. My family makes a whole weekend of it, and everyone goes home with a few jars for themselves. During the week, I'll come home, and simply cook some whole wheat pasta and toss it with pesto for an instant meal. Or I might stuff it under the skin of chicken breasts and bake them in the oven for twenty minutes. What could be easier? Or I might add a few flavorful spoonfuls to a vegetable soup.

When tomatoes are in season—ripe and delicious—Alan will buy a crate of them and I'll spend a day making "Candied" Tomatoes (page 76) and store them in olive oil in the refrigerator. They make a great Level Two lunch with cannellini beans, served atop a green salad, or a slice of grilled whole wheat bread with some fresh basil. A fast dinner is an omelet filled with "Candied" Tomatoes and caramelized onions. Grill a fresh fillet of sole and top it with "Candied" Tomatoes; it takes no more than ten minutes and is fit for company. Serve with lamb chops or chicken . . . I could go on and on.

I like to roast a chicken on Sundays for my family and serve it with vegetables and baked garlic. I'll bake some extra garlic and store it in the refrigerator for a quick lunch with sautéed vegetables or pasta. I'll remove all the leftover meat from the chicken and use it for a chicken salad or grilled with vegetables. Then I make from the carcass a rich, dark chicken stock that I use later on for vegetable soup, chicken soup, or as a flavoring in sauces.

So whenever you cook, constantly think ahead. In today's busy world, it's a wonderful treat to have in your freezer or refrigerator the fresh, delicious ingredients and components of an instant, healthy, and appetizing meal.

A Few Tips on Preparation

Steaming This is one of the easiest ways to enjoy fresh vegetables. It's best to have a steamer; but you can do it in a microwave, or on the stove with a removable steamer. I like to steam vegetables until they are still slightly crisp. When you stick a fork in the vegetables, it goes in easily but the vegetables are still firm. Different vegetables take different amounts of time to cook, so don't steam all your vegetables at once.

Pasta Do not overcook whole wheat pasta products—they turn to mush. Prepare according to package instructions and keep tasting until you get your desired firmness. Then drain and rinse in cold water to prevent sticking. Save a few spoonfuls of the water in which the pasta was cooked for use in your sauce.

Grilling One of my favorite ways to cook. I make everything on the grill, from vegetables to chicken breasts and fish to whole wheat bread. I love to cook outside in nice weather. I recently remodeled my kitchen so I also have an indoor grill. Or I can use grill pans that fit right over the burner. They're available at cooking stores, and are a lot less expensive than remodeling your kitchen. I like to use my outdoor gas grill so I don't have to worry about the potential health hazards of grilling over charcoal.

Seasoning I always like to season with fresh herbs. If you don't have space to grow herbs in a garden, basil, thyme, rosemary, sage, and parsley will grow just fine in a window garden. I love fried sage leaves sprinkled over cannellini beans. Fresh thyme is great over any kind of tomato or zucchini dish. Use fresh parsley over pasta or in sauces, or fresh rosemary with lamb. Sprinkle fresh parsley or basil into vegetable soup. If a window garden is not an option for you, then fill your spice cabinet with as many dried spices as possible.

In addition to herbs, I use salt, pepper, and lemon *liberally* to taste. On Level Two, I also sprinkle a little olive oil with a squeeze of fresh lemon, salt, and pepper on salads or pastas.

CHAPTER ELEVEN

Level One: Let's Get Cookin'

I developed the following recipes as a result of many trips to Europe, where I traveled through Italy and France. For example, the stuffed vegetables on pages 102–104 were inspired by my many visits to Saint-Tropez. I had them at a wonderful place called Café des Art, and then created a Somersize version, substituting mushrooms for bread crumbs in the filling—which I found was better than the original! When you prepare this recipe, you may find a substitute that's even better than mine. I always cook with fresh herbs, vegetables, and olive oil. I prefer the taste of olive oil to butter, and so my cooking is more Tuscan-based than French-based.

These are meals I enjoy making for my family members (who love the taste of these foods that keep them trim and healthy), and they are suitable for entertaining the fussiest of guests. These dishes will serve as a blueprint for the delicious meals ahead of you. In no time you will be creating your own recipes, all the while marveling at your newly shaped body and wondering how you could possibly have ever eaten any other way. You'll never feel deprived or hungry.

Good luck as you *eat great* and *lose weight!*

Dips, Spreads, and Appetizers

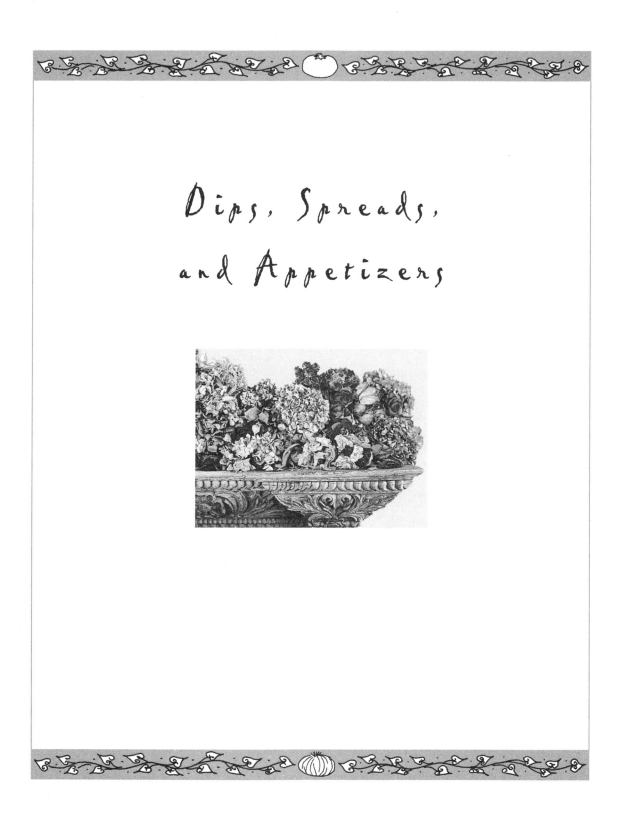

Cannellini Bean Dip

CARBOS AND VEGGIES; LEVEL ONE

MAKES 1 ½ CUPS

The wonderful flavor of cannellini beans with fresh sage reminds me of our summer vacations in Tuscany, Italy. That's where I first tasted them, and now they are part of my regular menus. I like them best with Roasted Red Peppers and Grilled Bread (page 81). This dip is also perfect when simply served with vegetables or used as a nonfat sandwich spread. For a lovely appetizer, try a dollop wrapped in red leaf lettuce with a tomato slice. Delicious!

3 cups cooked cannellini beans
   (or any other white beans)
1 garlic clove
Juice from 1 lemon

2 tablespoons chopped fresh sage
   (or parsley)
Salt and freshly ground black pepper

   Place all the ingredients in a food processor or blender. Puree until smooth. Adjust seasonings to taste, and add more lemon juice if desired.

For Level Two
Add 3 tablespoons extra-virgin olive oil for additional flavor and a smoother consistency. Top with toasted pine nuts. This addition of fat to your Carbos creates a small imbalance.

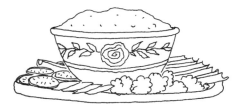

Baba Ganoush

VEGGIES; LEVEL ONE

❖

MAKES 1 1/2 CUPS

This is a delicious dip with whole wheat pita triangles and fresh vegetables. Grilling the eggplant adds a wonderful charred flavor. Also a great nonfat sandwich spread, the dip can be used instead of mayonnaise. Or try it on a piece of grilled chicken! Alan loves it.

1 large eggplant
Juice from 1 lemon

3 garlic cloves, chopped
5 to 8 dashes of Tabasco sauce

Place the eggplant on a prepared grill over medium heat, turning occasionally, until blackened and soft on all sides, about 30 minutes. (Or you can roast the eggplant in the oven on a baking sheet, turning often until the eggplant is roasted on all sides.)

Remove the eggplant from the heat. Immediately place it in a Ziploc bag, seal the bag, and let the eggplant steam for about 30 minutes. Remove the eggplant from the bag, peel off the skin and stem, and place the meat in a food processor. Add the remaining ingredients, puree, and adjust seasonings to taste.

For Level Two
Add 3 tablespoons tahini (sesame paste) and blend. The tahini, which is similar to peanut butter, adds flavor and smoothness.

"Candied" Tomatoes

SERVES 6

My husband, Alan, always buys too much food. He just can't help himself, especially when it comes to perfectly ripe fruits or vegetables. I devised this recipe one day when I was staring at a crate of ready-to-eat tomatoes on our kitchen table and realized there was no way the two of us could finish them before they died. I now make these tomatoes regularly and store them in olive oil in the refrigerator. What a treat! They have an incredible taste; if you cook nothing else from this book, make these "candied"-tasting tomatoes.

On Level One, make a terrific side dish by using these tomatoes in Vegetables Provençal (page 92); or spoon them over chicken breasts for a main course. The tomatoes are also great in omelets, sprinkled with fresh thyme leaves. On Level Two, serve warm with grilled bread (see page 81) and fresh basil leaves, or spoon over cannellini beans for a warm or cold al fresco lunch.

6 large ripe tomatoes
¼ cup olive oil
Salt

Preheat the oven to 325°F.

Slice the tomatoes in half crosswise. Place the tomatoes on a baking sheet, cut side up. Pour the oil over the tomatoes. Sprinkle with salt as desired. Bake for about 2 hours, until tomatoes are wrinkled on the outside but still somewhat moist in the center. Serve warm or cool.

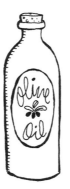

Hummus with Pita Triangles and Crudités

CARBOS AND VEGGIES; LEVEL ONE

SERVES 4

This is a delicious dip with whole wheat pita triangles and fresh vegetables. It's also a great nonfat sandwich spread instead of mayonnaise. Garbanzo beans can be purchased dried or canned, which are cooked and ready to use.

4 cups cooked or canned garbanzo beans (chickpeas)
3 garlic cloves
4 tablespoons lemon juice
Dash of cayenne pepper
1 sprig parsley

1 package whole wheat pita (4 pockets), cut into triangles
Assorted cut-up raw vegetables (broccoli, zucchini strips, radishes, red and green bell pepper slices)

In a food processor or blender, puree the garbanzos with the garlic, lemon juice, and cayenne until smooth. Adjust seasoning to taste. Garnish with a sprig of parsley and a sprinkle of cayenne. Spread on pita triangles and serve with crudités.

For Level Two
Blend in 2 tablespoons tahini (sesame paste) and garnish with toasted pine nuts.

Fat-Free Yogurt Dressings

CARBOS AND VEGGIES; LEVEL ONE

MAKES ENOUGH FOR ABOUT 4 SALADS

These tangy, light, delicious dressings have no fat, which makes them perfect salad toppers for Carbos and Veggies meals.

LEMON-MINT

1 cup plain nonfat yogurt
Juice from ½ lemon

12 fresh mint leaves
Salt and freshly ground black pepper

Combine all the ingredients in a blender or food processor and blend until smooth. Adjust seasonings to taste.

PIQUANT

1 cup plain nonfat yogurt
2 tablespoons salsa

In a bowl, combine all the ingredients using a fork. Adjust salsa to taste.

ROASTED RED PEPPER

1 cup plain nonfat yogurt
1 Roasted Red Pepper (page 81)

1 garlic clove
⅛ teaspoon cayenne
Salt and freshly ground black pepper

Combine all the ingredients in a blender or food processor and blend until smooth. Adjust seasonings to taste.

Basil Pesto

MAKES 1 CUP

Pesto is a staple in every Italian kitchen. I am never without it in my refrigerator. When I come home from a long trip, I always know I have a Level Two meal in the house if there's pasta in the pantry and a jar of pesto.

There are many, many ways to use pesto. Serve it over fresh tomatoes and buffalo mozzarella. A dollop of pesto is great on your favorite soup. Or try it as a topping for chicken or lamb. Pesto also makes a great roasted chicken—rub the pesto underneath the skin of the chicken so that the pesto is between the skin and the breast meat. Then rub the outside of the chicken with additional pesto before baking.

1 or more garlic cloves
3 tablespoons unsalted butter
¼ teaspoon ground white pepper
Pinch of freshly grated nutmeg
½ cup freshly grated Parmesan cheese
2 cups loosely packed basil leaves, stems
   removed

¼ cup flat-leaf parsley leaves, stems
   removed
¼ cup extra-virgin olive oil
Salt and freshly ground black pepper

To a food processor fitted with a steel blade, add the garlic, butter, white pepper, and nutmeg. With the processor running, add the Parmesan, then the basil and the parsley. Trickle the oil into the processor until the sauce is smooth. If necessary, add a little hot water to the sauce in order to reach the desired consistency. Then add salt and pepper to taste.

For Level Two
To the garlic, butter, pepper, and nutmeg, add 2 tablespoons walnuts and 1 tablespoon pine nuts. Prepare as above, and toss with some whole-grain pasta.

Baked Garlic

When baked, garlic becomes very sweet and spreads like butter. It's a great spread on chicken or lamb. It's also delicious with grilled vegetables like zucchini, eggplant, or mushrooms, and absolutely decadent as a dip for your favorite cheese, especially Stilton or Brie. The day after you eat this, your breath will smell so pungent that people entering a room will know instantly if you've been in it.

1 head of garlic per serving
Olive oil
Fresh or dried thyme

Preheat the oven to 350° F.

Slice the tops off the garlic heads, exposing the cluster of cloves. Brush with a touch of olive oil and sprinkle with thyme. Place in shallow baking pan and bake 45 minutes, or until golden brown and bubbly.

For Level One Carbos and Veggies Meal
Omitting the olive oil when preparing the garlic allows you to spread the baked garlic on Level One Carbos and Veggies foods. Try the garlic on a toasted pita with grilled vegetables.

For Level Two
Baked Garlic is at its absolute best when eaten with a bite of Stilton cheese. If you include bread along with the garlic and cheese, it will create an imbalance you will have to adjust to.

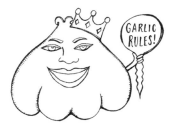

Roasted Red Peppers and Grilled Bread

CARBOS AND VEGGIES: LEVEL ONE

Roasted red peppers are great with everything, especially Baked Garlic (opposite). And since they are Veggies, they can also be served with Proteins/Fats. Try them with thinly sliced Pecorino cheese. Yum!

ROASTED RED PEPPERS

Red bell peppers (or your favorite color)

For the roasted peppers: Place the whole peppers on a prepared hot grill or an open flame and char on all sides until the skins are black and bubbling. Immediately put the roasted peppers into a Ziploc bag and seal. Let the peppers steam in the bag for 15 minutes. (This steaming process will make the peeling easier.)

Remove the peppers from the bag and pull the stems off. Break the peppers apart and discard the seeds. The charred skins will peel off easily. (I find it's faster to seed and peel the peppers under cool running water.) Break into strips and arrange on a platter.

GRILLED BREAD

Sliced whole-grain bread
Whole garlic cloves (1 per slice of bread)

For the grilled bread: Grill the bread over high heat, turning when nicely toasted on each side. While still warm, rub the bread with garlic. Serve with the roasted red peppers.

For Level Two

Drizzle olive oil on the bread before grilling.

Pickled Okra

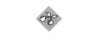

MAKES 8 PINTS

Pickling is quite a process, but it's a great way to prepare this underrated vegetable. I like crunchy okra with grilled meats, chicken, or turkey sausages. Or leave them out on the kitchen counter and see how quickly they are devoured. You will need eight 1-pint canning jars with lids and screw bands.

2 pounds tender young okra
1 quart white vinegar
3 cups water
6 tablespoons kosher salt
16 small garlic cloves, peeled

8 small fresh hot red peppers
8 whole cloves
1 bunch fresh dill
1 tablespoon pickling spices
½ cup mustard seeds

Rinse the okra and cut away any bruises or bad spots. Trim the stem ends but do not remove caps entirely.

To sterilize the canning jars, wash the jars, lids, and screw bands with hot, soapy water; rinse well. Place jars upright on a wire rack in a large pot. Fill pot with hot water until jars are submerged by 1 to 2 inches, and bring water to a boil. Boil for 15 minutes, then turn off heat. Sterilize lids according to manufacturer's instructions.

In a large pot, bring the vinegar, water, and salt to a boil.

Using stainless-steel tongs, remove the canning jars from the hot water and set on a layer of clean towels.

Evenly divide the garlic, peppers, cloves, dill sprigs, pickling spices, and mustard seeds and place in the jars. Pack tightly with the okra, alternating vertical direction of caps. Leave a ¾ inch space beneath the rim of the jar. Pour the hot vinegar liquid over the okra,

covering by ¼ inch and leaving ½ inch space below the rim. Slide a clean plastic chopstick or wooden skewer along the inside of each jar to release any air bubbles. Wipe the mouth of each jar with a clean, damp cloth. Place a hot lid on each jar, then add the screw band and turn firmly without forcing.

Using a jar lifter, place the jars on the rack in the large pot. Add enough additional hot water to cover by 2 inches, and bring to a boil. Boil jars for 10 minutes, then remove from water bath; let stand on a clean dish towel for 24 hours.

Check cooled jars for the slight indentation in the lids that indicates a vacuum seal. Jars that do not seal properly or that leak during processing should be stored in the refrigerator and the pickled okra consumed within a week. Allow sealed pickles to cool in a dry place for 6 to 8 weeks before serving. Store opened jars in the refrigerator.

Crispy Fried Eggplant and Mozzarella Finger Sandwiches

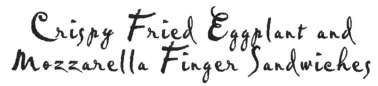

PROTEINS/FATS AND VEGGIES; LEVEL ONE

MAKES ABOUT 20 FINGER SANDWICHES

Alan asks for these often. I feel like I'm cheating when I eat them, because they taste so good. Serve them hot off the stove or over baby greens tossed with Balsamic Vinaigrette (page 106) for a great salad. (You can cook these a few hours in advance and reheat at serving time, if you like.)

SANDWICHES

4 Japanese eggplants, sliced slightly on the diagonal into ½-inch-thick slices
2 to 3 tablespoons olive oil
Salt and freshly ground black pepper

1 pound fresh mozzarella cheese, cut into ¼-inch-thick slices
3 large eggs, lightly beaten
1 cup freshly grated Parmesan cheese
Vegetable oil, for frying

HERB SPREAD

3 garlic cloves
½ cup loosely packed basil leaves
¼ cup loosely packed flat-leaf parsley
⅛ teaspoon hot red pepper flakes
3 tablespoons olive oil

Preheat the oven to 425°F.

For the sandwiches: On a baking sheet, lightly brush the eggplant slices with olive oil; season with salt and pepper. Bake for 15 minutes, until golden brown. Set aside.

For the herb spread: In a food processor, combine the garlic, basil, parsley, red pepper flakes, and oil. Blend until well combined.

Spread the paste on half of the roasted eggplant slices, then top each of the paste-covered slices with a piece of mozzarella. (You may need to trim the cheese to fit the shape of the eggplant.) Make little finger sandwiches by placing the remaining eggplant pieces on top of the cheese.

Dip each finger sandwich in the beaten egg, then in the Parmesan cheese, until well coated. Heat ½ inch of vegetable oil in a sauté pan. (The oil should be about 350°F. for best results.) Sauté the finger sandwiches for a couple minutes on each side, until nicely browned. Drain on paper towels. You will need to cook the sandwiches in batches, reserving the cooked ones in a warm oven.

Tuscan Deep-Fried Artichokes

PROTEINS/FATS AND VEGGIES; LEVEL ONE

SERVES 4

These are like french fries made of artichokes.

4 large artichokes
Juice from 1 lemon

Salt and freshly ground black pepper
2 quarts (or more) vegetable oil, for frying

Clean the artichokes by trimming off the bottom stalks and removing the tough outer leaves. To prevent discoloration, reserve artichokes as they are prepared in a bowl of water with the lemon juice. When all the artichokes are trimmed, drain them and pat dry. Pull the leaves apart to slightly expose the center. Sprinkle the inside and between the leaves as best you can with salt and pepper.

Heat the oil in a deep pot until it reaches 350°F. (A candy thermometer is helpful.)

The key is to have the oil at the right temperature so that the artichokes cook on the inside without burning on the outside. Add the artichokes to the oil and cook for approximately 10 minutes, or until crisp and golden. (You may need to cook them in batches, depending on the size of your pot.) Turn them often, pressing them against the bottom of the pan with a utensil to open the leaves. When cooked, drain on paper towels. Sprinkle again with salt and pepper and serve immediately.

Steamed Artichokes with Lemon-Dill Mayonnaise

PROTEINS/FATS AND VEGGIES; LEVEL ONE

SERVES 4

Nothing is as delicious as a beautifully presented artichoke for lunch or dinner. Slowly eating this delightful treat is a great way to sit and talk with guests. Serve artichokes hot or cold with my wonderful Lemon-Dill Mayonnaise for dipping. I also like steamed artichokes with Garlic Vinaigrette (page 95).

Juice from 2 lemons
4 large artichokes

1 teaspoon celery seeds
1 teaspoon dried dill

Place the lemon juice in a bowl of water. Trim the artichokes by cutting off the stalks and removing the tough outer leaves. Slice about ½ of the artichoke off the top, cutting off inedible, prickly leaves and barely exposing the purple center or choke. Trim the tips off any remaining prickly leaves with scissors. Reserve the prepared artichokes in the bowl of lemon water to prevent discoloration.

Place about 4 inches of water, celery seeds, and dill in the bottom of a steamer. Place the artichokes in the steamer basket and steam until tender. Cooking time will vary depending on the size of the artichoke, from 40 to 60 minutes.

Lemon-Dill Mayonnaise

MAKES ABOUT ¹/₂ CUP

1 recipe Homemade Mayonnaise (page 86)
    or prepared mayonnaise
Juice from 1 lemon

1 tablespoon finely chopped fresh dill
    or 2 teaspoons dried dill
Freshly ground black pepper

Combine all the ingredients in a bowl and adjust seasonings to your taste.

Homemade Mayonnaise

PROTEINS/FATS; LEVEL ONE

MAKES 1 1/2 CUPS

Mizou, my daughter-in-law's mother, always makes her own mayonnaise for salads, shellfish, and vegetables. Homemade mayonnaise has a smooth, silky texture that you won't find in store-bought versions. It takes only a couple of minutes to make and will last for about a week in the refrigerator. To make an herbed mayonnaise, add your favorite freshly chopped herbs, such as dill, tarragon, chives, or basil. Serve as a dip or sauce with hot or cold veggies.

2 large organic eggs (see Note)
1 teaspoon red wine vinegar
Juice from 1/2 lemon
1/2 teaspoon salt

1/4 teaspoon ground white pepper
Dash of Tabasco sauce
Dash of Worcestershire sauce
1 cup vegetable oil

Combine all the ingredients except the oil in a bowl. Blend with a whisk, or in a blender. Add the oil very gradually in a thin stream, whisking constantly. Adjust seasonings to taste and refrigerate.

Note Wash fresh eggs in shells in soapy water first and rinse thoroughly to help avoid any danger of salmonella.

Chicken Drummettes

MAKES ABOUT 30 DRUMMETTES

These chicken drummettes are great appetizers. Prepare plenty because they get gobbled up quickly!

2 pounds chicken drummettes
⅓ cup olive oil
Juice from 3 lemons
10 garlic cloves, pressed
10 sprigs fresh thyme leaves

1 bunch flat-leaf parsley, chopped
1 tablespoon dried rosemary
½ teaspoon or more cayenne pepper
1 teaspoon paprika
Salt and freshly ground black pepper

Combine all the ingredients in a noncorrosive bowl. Let marinate for 1 hour or more.

Heat a grill until very hot. Place the drummettes on the grill and cook for about 10 minutes, turning constantly. They should become nicely charred from the olive oil in the marinade. (If you do not like them charred, lower the heat to medium.)

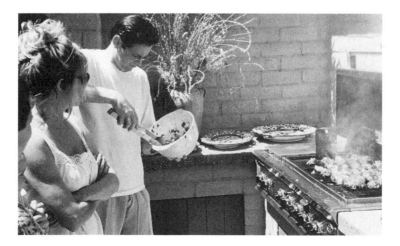

My son Bruce cooking Chicken Drummettes.

Fruit Smoothie

SERVES 2

Alan makes breakfast; I make dinner. That's what works in our marriage. I don't wake up easily in the morning until Alan taps me gently on the shoulder with one of these delicious fruit smoothies. Experiment with various combinations of fruit (except bananas). This one is particularly yummy.

1 mango, peeled and seeded
1 papaya, peeled and seeded
½ cup fresh raspberries

¾ cup orange juice
Strawberries, for garnish
A few ice cubes, if desired

Place the fruit and orange juice in a blender and process until smooth. Adjust the amount of juice to create the consistency you prefer. If you like your smoothie frozen, use frozen fruit or add a few ice cubes. Serve in wineglasses with a strawberry garnish.

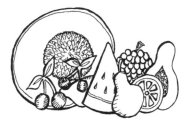

Side Dishes (That Can Make a Meal)

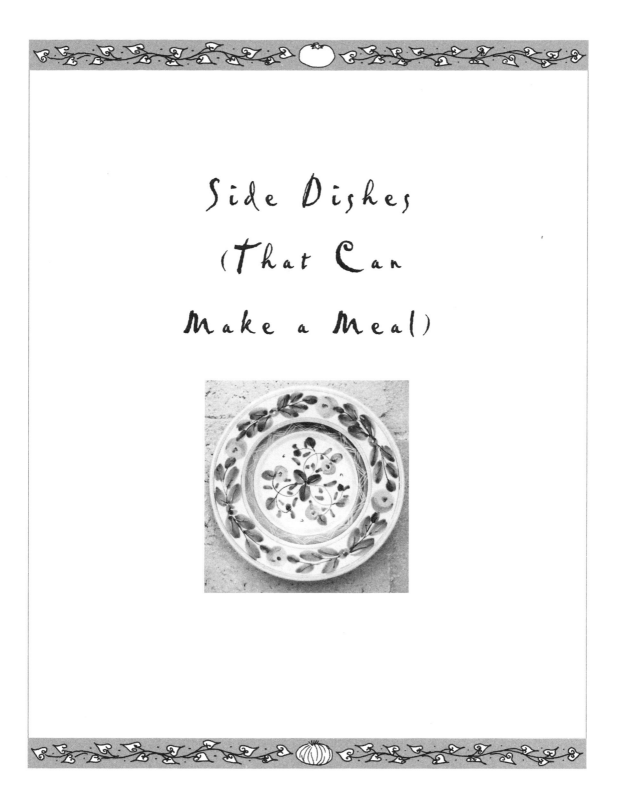

Grilled Zucchini and Eggplant

PROTEINS/FATS AND VEGGIES; LEVEL ONE

SERVES 6

You can make these on an indoor grill or an outdoor barbecue. The thinner you slice the veggies, the better. The small amount of olive oil really brings out the taste of the vegetables; they are great tasting, satisfying, and won't add an inch to your waistline. Serve the vegetables with any of your favorite protein dishes.

6 medium zucchini
6 Japanese eggplants

A few tablespoons olive oil
Salt and freshly ground black pepper

Preheat the grill to high.

Slice the zucchini and eggplants lengthwise as thin as possible. (A mandolin is very helpful.) Place the slices on a hot grill and brush with a very small amount of olive oil. Turn quickly when charred. The thinner the slices, the faster the cooking time. Sprinkle with salt and pepper and arrange on a platter to serve, alternating the zucchini and the eggplant.

**For Level One Carbos
and Veggies Meal**
Omit the olive oil when preparing the vegetables. Serve with Roasted Red Peppers and Grilled Bread (page 81) for a delicious treat.

Summer Squash Medley

SERVES 4 TO 6

My son Bruce has always loved vegetables . . . lots of them. Except squash. I started making this for him when he was a little boy; it was the only way I could get him to eat this particular vegetable. He still asks for this dish, even though he's now thirty. The difference is, he no longer has to finish his squash to get to stay up late.

2 medium zucchini
2 medium crookneck squash
2 pattypan squash
2 tablespoons olive oil

1 teaspoon dried dill
Salt and freshly ground black pepper
Juice from 1 lemon

Slice the zucchini lengthwise and then chop crosswise, creating half-moon slices. Repeat with the crookneck squash. Quarter the pattypan squash and cut the quarters into half-moon slices as well.

Heat a wok or skillet over high heat. Add the olive oil and squash. Sprinkle with the dill, salt, pepper, and lemon juice. Sauté quickly for 5 to 8 minutes, or until tender.

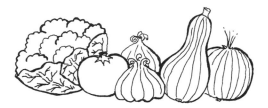

Vegetables Provençal

SERVES 6

This combination of flavors will make any meal a sensation! Try it with your favorite meat, poultry, or fish. It may seem like a lot of onions to start with, but they cook down quite a bit and have an intense flavor when they caramelize.

⅓ cup olive oil
3 medium onions, sliced
5 garlic cloves, thinly sliced
3 medium zucchini, sliced

8 sprigs fresh thyme leaves
Salt and freshly ground black pepper
12 "Candied" Tomatoes (page 76)

Heat the olive oil in a large skillet. Add the onions and cook over medium-low heat until browned and caramelized, about 30 minutes. Add the garlic and cook for 1 minute. Turn up the heat to medium high and add the zucchini (and additional oil if the pan seems too dry). Cook until tender, about 8 minutes. Sprinkle with thyme leaves, salt, and pepper. Add the tomatoes and stir until combined. Continue cooking until the tomatoes are heated through, about 5 minutes.

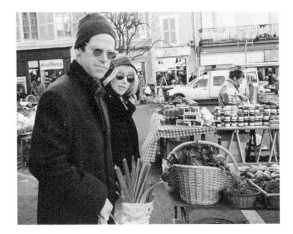

With my stepson Stephen, shopping for Christmas dinner at the open-air market in Montélimar, France.

Zucchini Carpaccio

PROTEINS/FATS AND VEGGIES; LEVEL ONE

SERVES 6

This is a beautiful lunch dish or first course. I serve it often on hot summer days at my home in the desert.

3 bunches arugula
⅓ cup extra-virgin olive oil
2 lemons

Salt and freshly ground black pepper
3 medium zucchini
Shavings of Parmesan cheese

Slice the zucchini lengthwise as thin as possible. (A mandolin is helpful.) Rinse and dry the arugula. Drizzle a little of the olive oil over the arugula, then squeeze the juice from 1 lemon on top. Toss with salt and pepper. Arrange the arugula on 6 plates.

Place the raw zucchini slices in a single layer over the arugula to cover it completely. Drizzle the zucchini with a little more olive oil and juice from the remaining lemon. Sprinkle with salt and pepper, then top with Parmesan cheese.

Squashed Pattypan Squash

PROTEINS/FATS AND VEGGIES; LEVEL ONE

SERVES 4

Squash is a delicious and satisfying food that is often overlooked. I like to serve this as a side-dish substitute for potatoes or other starch. I suggest three garlic cloves in this recipe, but Alan likes me to double up and add six. If you do this, share the dish with someone you love.

6 pattypan squash, quartered
3 garlic cloves, smashed
1 tablespoon olive oil

½ cup water
1 tablespoon butter
Salt and freshly ground black pepper

In a small saucepan, place the squash, garlic, and olive oil. Add the water and cover. Bring to a boil, then reduce heat and simmer for 5 to 7 minutes.

Remove from the heat and drain off the water. Remove the garlic and add the butter. Smash with a fork until chunky. Season with salt and pepper.

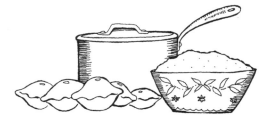

Green Beans with Garlic Vinaigrette

PROTEINS/FATS AND VEGGIES; LEVEL ONE

SERVES 4

Have you noticed? I love the flavor of garlic. It's also very good for you. This dish is delicious hot or cold, and the vinaigrette is also good on salads or other vegetables.

1 pound fresh green beans
Garlic Vinaigrette (recipe follows)

   Steam the beans until tender and still slightly crunchy; don't overcook. Toss with vinaigrette and serve.

Garlic Vinaigrette

MAKES 1/4 CUP

2 to 3 garlic cloves, pressed
Juice from 1 lemon

Salt and freshly ground black pepper
¼ cup extra-virgin olive oil

   Mix the garlic, lemon juice, salt, and pepper in a bowl. In a slow stream, whisk in the olive oil until combined.

Sautéed Fennel

PROTEINS/FATS AND VEGGIES; LEVEL ONE

SERVES 6

Fennel is an underrated and underused vegetable, which I discovered on one of my many trips to France. It has a wonderfully subtle flavor and makes a tasty side dish to your favorite meat, poultry, or fish.

2 fennel bulbs
3 tablespoons olive oil
Salt and freshly ground black pepper

Remove the tops of the fennel until just the bulb remains. Slice the bulbs into ¼-inch-thick pieces. Heat the olive oil in a large skillet and add the fennel. Sauté for about 8 minutes. Season to taste with salt and pepper.

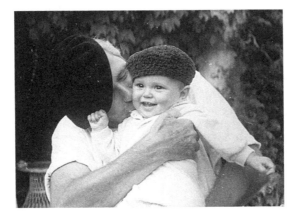

*Alan and our granddaughter
on vacation in Saint-Tropez. Very French!*

Japanese Eggplant and Chinese Long Beans with Ginger Soy Sauce

PROTEINS/FATS AND VEGGIES; LEVEL ONE

❦

SERVES 8 AS A SIDE DISH, 4 AS A MAIN DISH

Asian seasonings are a great way to flavor vegetables and give them a new twist. My daughter-in-law Caroline, who's an amazing cook, gave me this recipe, which can be served hot or cold.

VEGETABLES

3 Japanese eggplants
1 pound Chinese long beans
4 tablespoons olive oil

1 bunch green onions, sliced on the
  diagonal
1 bunch chives, chopped into 2-inch pieces

SAUCE

1 tablespoon grated fresh ginger
6 tablespoons soy sauce
2 tablespoons rice vinegar

Freshly ground black pepper
Hot red pepper flakes

For the vegetables: Trim the stems from the eggplants and slice them lengthwise in half. Trim the ends of the green beans.

Heat a large sauté pan over high heat. Add 2 tablespoons of the olive oil, then the eggplant and cook until brown and soft, about 5 minutes on each side. Using tongs, transfer the eggplant to a platter, reserving any liquid in the pan. Add another tablespoon of olive oil and the long beans to the pan, cooking until just tender, about 5 minutes. Remove the beans and place on the platter with the eggplant.

For the sauce: Reduce heat to low. Add the last tablespoon of olive oil and the ginger to the liquid in the pan from the vegetables. Sauté until golden, about 3 minutes. Add the soy sauce, rice vinegar, a few grindings of black pepper, and just a pinch of red pepper flakes.

Place the eggplant and beans back in the pan and coat with the sauce. Toss in the green onions and chives.

For Level Two
Serve the vegetables over brown rice for a great entrée.

Celery Root Puree

SERVES 6

While it looks like an old horse's hoof when it's uncooked, celery root has a wonderful, subtle flavor when it's peeled and pureed. In this recipe it makes a great substitute for mashed potatoes.

3 celery roots
¼ cup heavy cream (optional)

4 tablespoons butter (or ¼ cup olive oil)
Salt and freshly ground black pepper

Place about 5 cups of water in a large pot fitted with a steamer and a lid. Bring to a boil.

Chop off the roots and peel off the outside layer of skin from the celery roots, being careful to remove all the brown. Cut each celery root into about 12 pieces, and place pieces in the steamer. Steam until very soft when poked with a fork, about 20 minutes.

Transfer the celery root to a food processor. Add the cream and butter and puree until smooth. (If you don't have a food processor, you can use an electric mixer.) Add additional cream or butter to achieve desired consistency, or, for a healthier option, omit the butter and cream and use a little olive oil instead. Sprinkle with salt and pepper.

Shredded Brussels Sprouts with Lime

PROTEINS/FATS AND VEGGIES; LEVEL ONE

SERVES 12 TO 14

Hate Brussels sprouts? You won't anymore. Just make sure you don't overcook them when you are sautéing. I serve these with Thanksgiving dinner, and they are a true crowd pleaser.

3 pounds Brussels sprouts
½ cup butter (or olive oil)

Juice from 3 to 4 limes
Salt and freshly ground black pepper

Cut the sprouts in half and lay flat on a chopping block. Cut each half into julienned strips.

Heat a large skillet over medium-high heat. Melt the butter, then add the sprouts and sauté until tender, about 6 to 10 minutes. Season with lime juice, salt, and pepper.

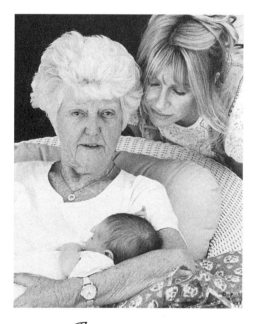

Three generations

Stir-Fried Vegetables

PROTEINS/FATS AND VEGGIES; LEVEL ONE

SERVES 4

Serve as a side dish, or add your favorite meat in the stir-fry along with the veggies.

2 tablespoons canola oil
6 cups coarsely chopped vegetables (baby
    bok choy, broccoli, snow peas, celery,
    onion, yellow squash)
5 to 10 dashes of soy sauce

Juice from 1 lemon
1 teaspoon toasted sesame oil
A few drops of chili oil
    (or ½ teaspoon hot red pepper flakes)

Place a wok or large frying pan over high heat. Add a little canola oil. Add the vegetables in small batches and cook quickly so the wok stays hot. As each batch is cooked, reserve vegetables on a platter until all are cooked (tender when poked with a fork, but not soggy).

Put all the vegetables back in the wok or frying pan and add the soy sauce, lemon juice, sesame oil, and chili oil or red pepper flakes.

For Level Two
Serve the vegetables over brown rice. This combination of oil and brown rice creates a slight imbalance.

Ratatouille

SERVES 8

Ratatouille is great hot or cold, alone or with chicken, beef, or fish. Make this in advance and keep it in the refrigerator for quick meals.

⅓ cup plus 2 tablespoons olive oil
2 medium onions, thinly sliced
2 garlic cloves
1 can (28 ounces) peeled tomatoes,
   with juice

4 bell peppers, julienned
Salt and freshly ground black pepper
1 large eggplant, peeled and diced
3 medium zucchini, cut into ½-inch slices

Heat a large, deep skillet over medium heat. Add ⅓ cup of the oil and the onion. Sauté until translucent. Add the garlic and cook for 1 more minute. Remove onion and garlic from the pan and set aside.

Quarter the tomatoes, reserving any juice. Set aside. Layer the bottom of the skillet with the peppers, salt and pepper, and ¼ of the onion-garlic mixture. Then layer with the eggplant, more salt and pepper, and another ¼ of the onion-garlic mixture. Repeat the layers using the zucchini, then the tomatoes in place of the eggplant and

finally topping with the remaining onion-garlic mixture. Pour in the reserved tomato juice and top with remaining 2 tablespoons of oil. Cover and simmer over very low heat for 35 to 40 minutes. Uncover and cook an additional 10 minutes to reduce the liquid.

For Level One Carbos and Veggies Meal
Omit the olive oil. Sauté the onion and garlic in a little tomato juice. Prepare as above and serve over whole-grain pasta or brown rice.

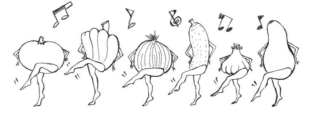

Stuffed Zucchini

PROTEINS/FATS AND VEGGIES; LEVEL ONE

MAKES 12 STUFFED ZUCCHINI; SERVES 6

My uncle Dave used to make these for us when we went to his house for dinner. Recently, I found out this wasn't his recipe at all but his wife's, my aunt Helen. Anyway, I added the red pepper flakes and sometimes have these as a yummy entrée with a green salad. It's like an Italian frittata sitting in a zucchini boat.

6 medium zucchini
2 tablespoons olive oil
1 medium onion, chopped
1 red bell pepper, chopped
3 garlic cloves, minced
Salt and freshly ground black pepper

Pinch of hot red pepper flakes (optional)
1 teaspoon dried oregano
2 large eggs, lightly beaten
1 tablespoon grated Parmesan cheese
1 teaspoon chopped fresh thyme leaves

Preheat the oven to 350°F.

Bring a large pot of salted water to a boil. Parboil the zucchini for 5 minutes, then remove from the water and let cool. Slice the zucchini in half lengthwise and scoop out the insides, creating a bowl to hold the stuffing. Reserve the zucchini insides in a medium bowl.

Heat a medium frying pan over high heat. Add the olive oil, onion, and red pepper. Sauté until the onion is transparent and the pepper is soft and slightly browned, about 5 minutes. Add the garlic and sauté 1 minute longer. Remove from the heat and add to the reserved zucchini. Season with salt, pepper, red pepper flakes, and oregano. Add the beaten eggs and blend the mixture, mashing the zucchini well.

Fill the zucchini shells with equal parts of the stuffing. Sprinkle with Parmesan cheese, pepper, and thyme. Place in an ungreased shallow baking dish and bake for 35 minutes, until stuffing is golden brown and bubbly. Serve immediately.

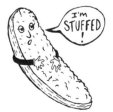

Stuffed Tomatoes

MAKES 12 STUFFED TOMATOES; SERVES 6

I vacation in Saint-Tropez every summer. These tomatoes are my version of the delicious Provençal treat that is a specialty of the area.

12 firm, ripe tomatoes
4 tablespoons olive oil
3 medium onions, thinly sliced
6 garlic cloves, finely chopped
8 ounces shiitake mushrooms, chopped
1 pound ground chicken or turkey
1 teaspoon fresh thyme leaves

1 tablespoon chopped fresh tarragon
1 bunch flat-leaf parsley, chopped
½ cup chicken broth
2 large eggs, beaten
2 tablespoons grated Parmesan cheese
Salt and freshly ground black pepper

Preheat the oven to 350° F.

Slice off the blossom end of each tomato and hollow out the insides with a small spoon. Set aside.

Heat a large saucepan over medium heat. Add the olive oil and onions. Sauté the onions until browned and caramelized, about 10 minutes. Add the garlic and sauté for 1 minute longer. Add the mushrooms and sauté until browned. Add the ground meat, ½ teaspoon of the thyme, the tarragon, and the parsley. Cook 5 to 10 minutes longer, or until the chicken is lightly browned. Then add the chicken broth and cook an additional 5 minutes. Remove the stuffing from the heat and place in a mixing bowl. Add the eggs and mix thoroughly with your hands.

Rub the inside of a shallow baking dish with olive oil. Fill the tomatoes with equal parts of the stuffing. Top each tomato with Parmesan cheese, the rest of the chopped thyme, a sprinkling of salt and pepper, and a drizzle of olive oil. Bake for 35 minutes or until the tomatoes are soft to the touch, basting occasionally with the pan juices. (If the juices evaporate too quickly, add a little water to the bottom of the pan.)

Spoon the pan juices over the stuffed tomatoes and serve immediately.

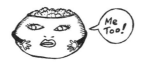

Side Dishes (That Can Make a Meal)

Stuffed Onions

MAKES 6 STUFFED ONIONS

These onions are inspired by a delicious dish I tasted in Saint-Tropez, but they're my own creation. As a main course, I serve a platter containing stuffed onions, tomatoes, and zucchini, beautifully arranged in the traditional Provençal way.

6 yellow or sweet onions
Salt and freshly ground black pepper
2 cups Mushroom Sausage Stuffing
  (page 167)
1 cup chicken broth
2 tablespoons grated Parmesan cheese

1 teaspoon fresh thyme leaves
  (or 1 teaspoon dried)
1 tablespoon chopped fresh tarragon
  (or 1 teaspoon dried)
Drizzle of olive oil

Preheat the oven to 350°F.

Peel each onion, then cut off the top quarter and scoop out the center until hollow. (Reserve the insides to sauté for stuffing or other use.) Season the onions inside and out with salt and pepper. Fill with stuffing and place in a shallow baking dish. Pour the chicken broth around the onions. Sprinkle the Parmesan cheese, thyme, and tarragon on the onions and drizzle a little olive oil on top. Bake for 30 minutes, or until tender and broth has reduced by half. Spoon the reduced broth over the onions and serve.

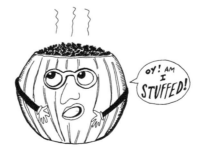

Whole Wheat Pasta with a classic sauce made from tomatoes at the peak of their flavor (page 145).

Minted Lamb in
Cucumber Boats with
Marinated Red Onion
(page 180) and my
beloved desert
in the background.

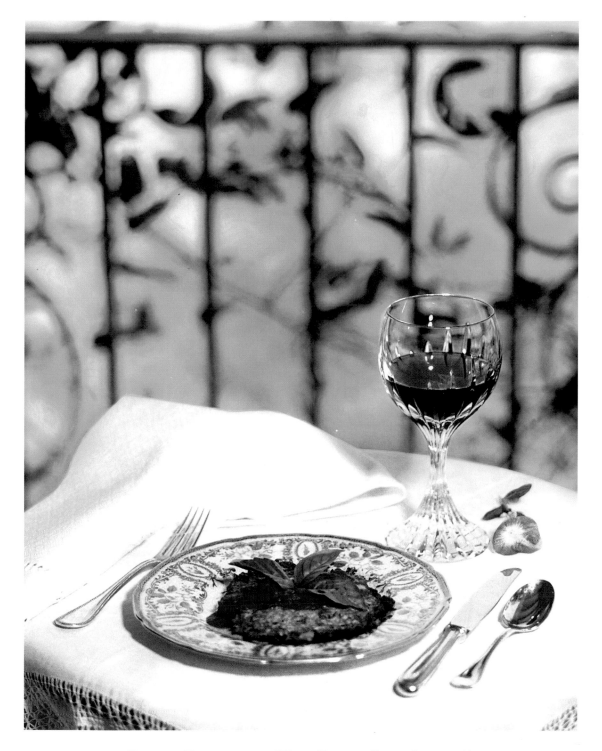

Zucchini Pancakes with Warm Tomato Coulis (page 140)

and one of my beautiful Irish linen tablecloths.

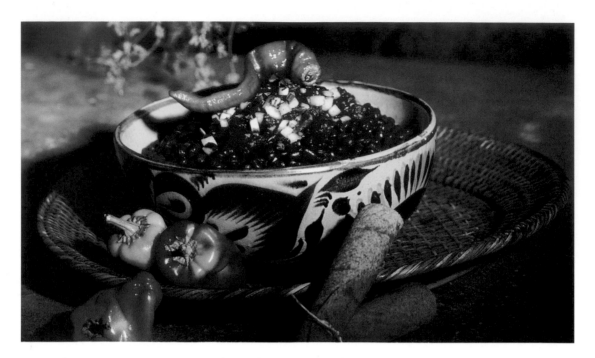

Black Bean Chili with Spicy Tomato Salsa (page 143).

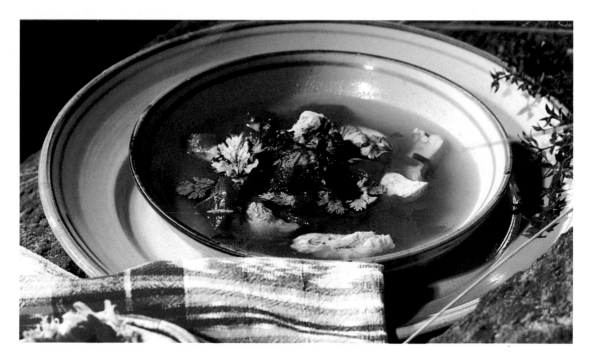

Chicken Tomato Cilantro Soup (page 126).

Yum!
Steaming hot
Whole Wheat
Popovers
(page 193).

Thanksgiving, the Somersize way, including turkey with mushroom sausage stuffing (page 166), pureed celery root (page 98), and green beans with vinaigrette (page 95).

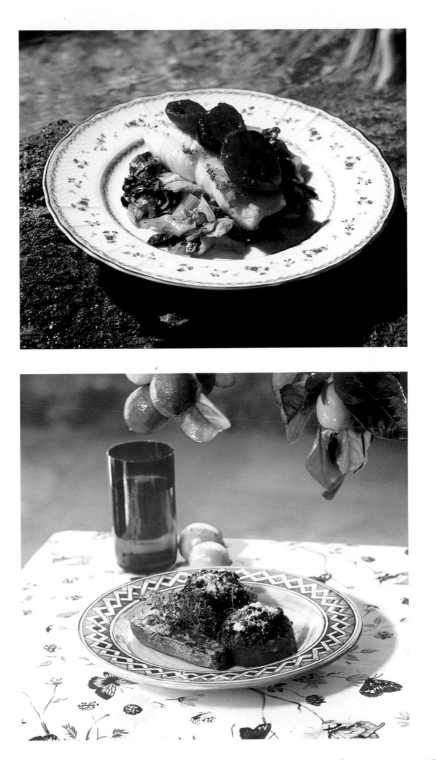

Top: Broiled Sea Bass with "Candied" Tomatoes and Seared Escarole (page 151).

Above: Stuffed vegetables—zucchini, tomatoes, and onions (pages 102—104).

Grilled bread with roasted red peppers (page 81) and baked garlic (page 80) make a fabulous Tuscan lunch.

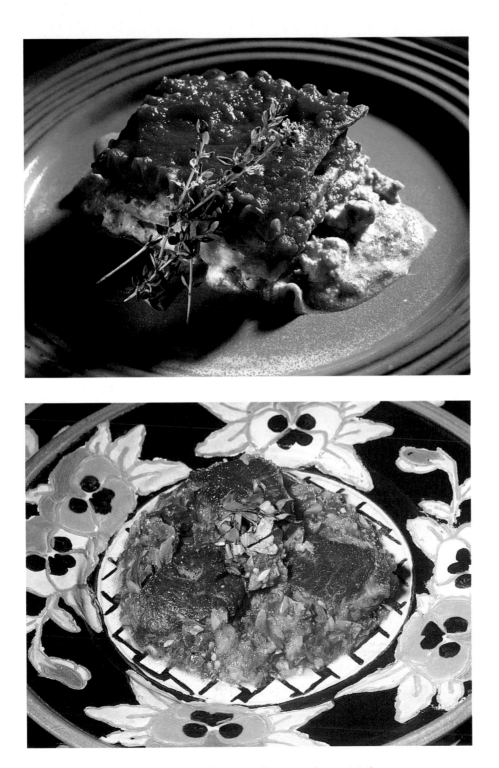

Top: Roasted Vegetable Lasagne (page 144).

Above: Medallions of Lamb in a tomato-basil sauce (page 178).

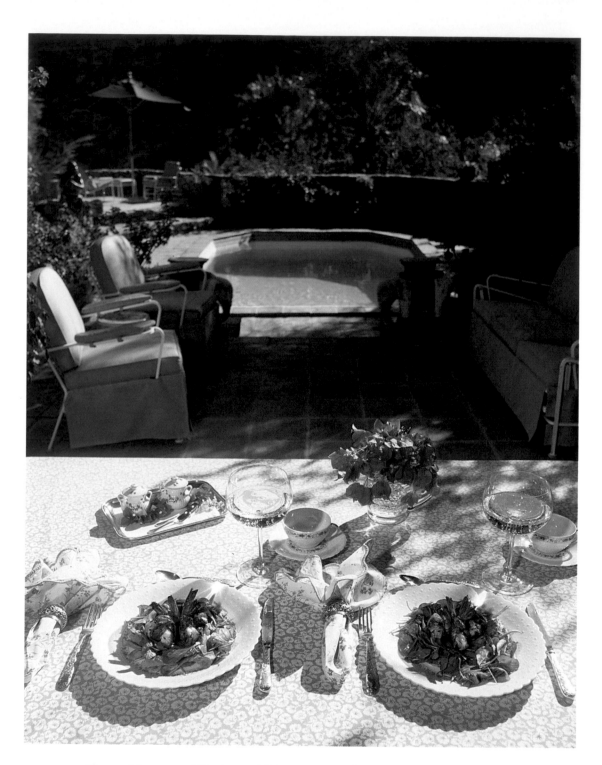

Citrus-Marinated Barbecued Shrimp with Fresh Arugula (page 148)—
perfect on a hot, summer desert day.

Every once in a while, it's fun to be a little crazy: a warm bath of rose petals while sipping a frosty Fruit Smoothie (page 88).

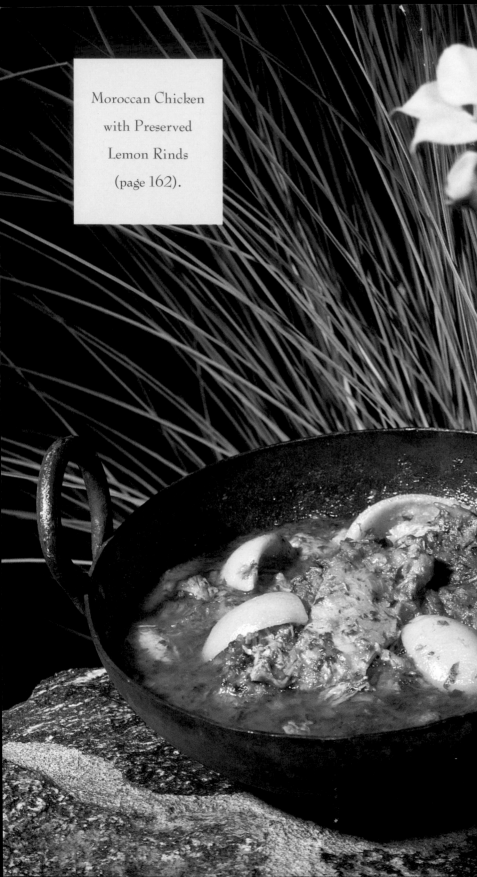

Moroccan Chicken
with Preserved
Lemon Rinds
(page 162).

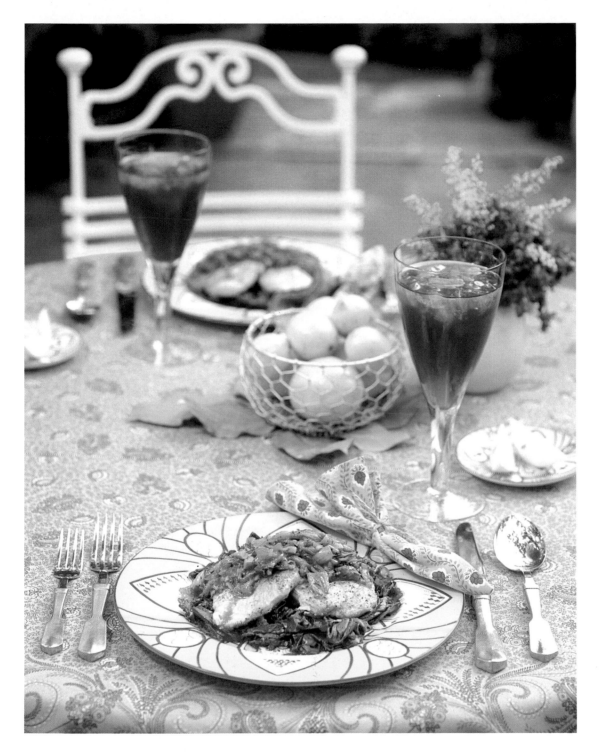

Chicken Paillard with Lemon-Parsley Butter and Seared Red Chard (page 160).

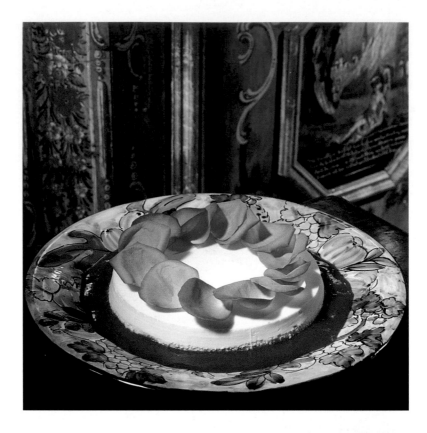

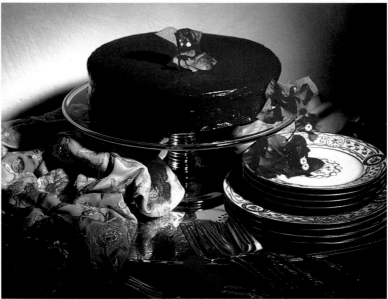

Top: Scrumptious Sugarless Cheesecake (page 186).

Above: My incredible Decadent Chocolate Cake (page 200).

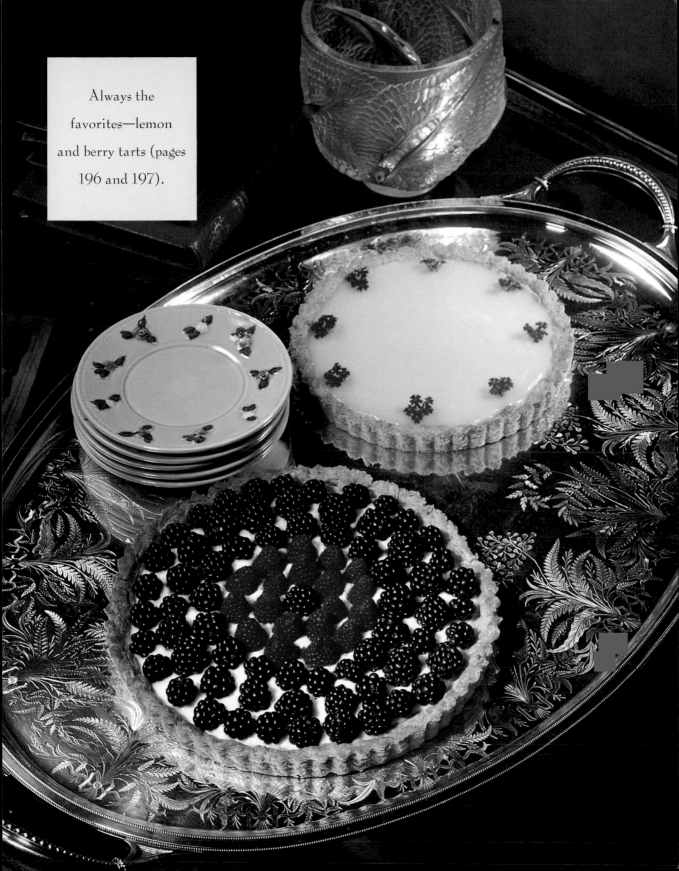

Always the favorites—lemon and berry tarts (pages 196 and 197).

At the end of the day,
what could be more
relaxing than sipping
ginger tea while
nibbling on fresh fruit,
surrounded by
beautiful lace?

Salads

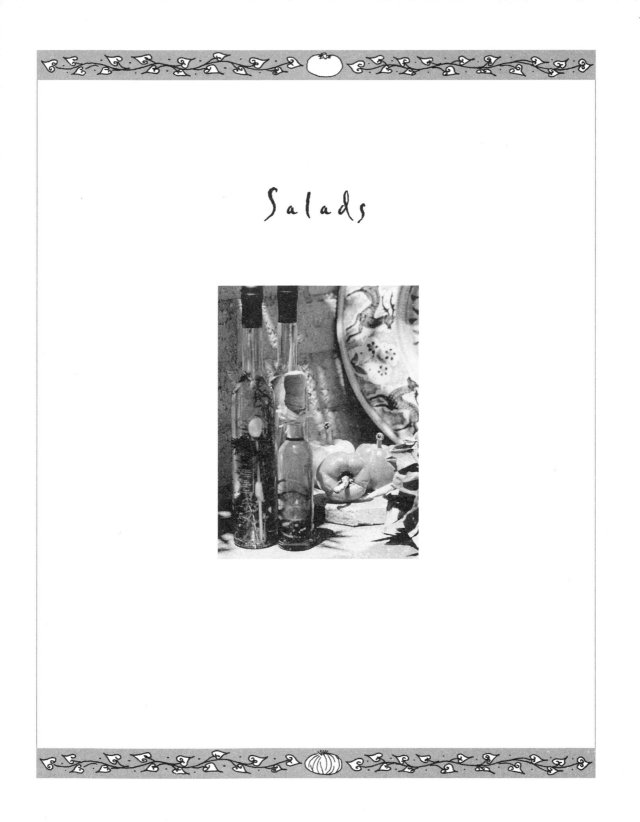

Tricoloré Salad with Balsamic Vinaigrette

PROTEINS/FATS AND VEGGIES; LEVEL ONE

SERVES 4 AS AN ENTRÉE OR 8 TO 10 AS A STARTER

When I was growing up, I had never heard of balsamic vinegar. Now it is one of the staples in my kitchen. This is a great, all-purpose salad to serve alone as lunch (topped with fresh shaved Parmesan) or as a first course with any dinner entrée.

1 pound mixed lettuce (radicchio, arugula, endive, or other), rinsed and dried

Balsamic Vinaigrette (recipe follows)
Salt and freshly ground black pepper

Tear the lettuces into medium pieces. You should have 8 cups loosely packed. Place the lettuces in a large bowl and toss with the vinaigrette just before serving. Season with salt and pepper.

Balsamic Vinaigrette

MAKES ABOUT 1/2 CUP

2 tablespoons balsamic vinegar
Salt and freshly ground black pepper
6 tablespoons olive oil

Place the vinegar in a mixing cup with salt and pepper to taste. Add the olive oil in a slow stream, constantly whisking until the oil is emulsified. For a tangier dressing, add more balsamic vinegar.

Green Salad with Artichoke Hearts and Red Wine Vinaigrette

PROTEINS/FATS AND VEGGIES; LEVEL ONE

SERVES 4 AS AN ENTRÉE OR 8 TO 10 AS A STARTER

Beautiful lettuce, delicious marinated artichoke hearts, a tangy vinaigrette ... perfection!

1 pound assorted lettuces (red leaf, butter, romaine), rinsed and dried
1 jar (8 ounces) marinated artichoke hearts, drained

½ medium red onion, chopped
Red Wine Vinaigrette (recipe follows)
Salt and freshly ground black pepper

Tear the lettuce into medium pieces and toss with the artichoke hearts, onion, and vinaigrette. Season with salt and pepper. Serve immediately.

Red Wine Vinaigrette

MAKES ABOUT ½ CUP

2 tablespoons red wine vinegar
1 teaspoon dried dill

Salt and freshly ground black pepper
6 tablespoons olive oil

Whisk together all the ingredients except the olive oil. Add the oil in a slow stream, whisking constantly until the oil is emulsified. For a tangier dressing, add more vinegar.

Iceberg Lettuce with Roquefort Dressing

PROTEINS/FATS AND VEGGIES; LEVEL ONE

SERVES 6

Sometimes the simplest salads taste the best. Try this delicious blue cheese dressing on any of your favorite lettuces.

1 head iceberg lettuce, rinsed and dried
Roquefort Dressing (recipe follows)

1 basket cherry tomatoes
Freshly ground black pepper

Slice the lettuce into thin strips. Arrange on 4 plates. Pour dressing over lettuce and garnish with cherry tomatoes. Season to taste with pepper.

Roquefort Dressing

MAKES ABOUT 1 1/2 CUPS

1 tablespoon red wine vinegar
4 ounces crumbled blue cheese,
  preferably Roquefort

¾ cup sour cream
Salt and freshly ground black pepper

Combine the ingredients in a food processor and blend until well mixed. (If you do not have a food processor, blend the ingredients in a bowl with a whisk until well mixed. I do not recommend putting this dressing in a blender because it is too thick.) If the dressing is too thick for your liking, add more vinegar until you reach the desired consistency.

Hearts of Palm Salad

SERVES 4

My son, Bruce, created this yummy salad, and now it's a family favorite.

1 can (14 ounces) hearts of palm, drained
 and chopped
6 celery stalks, chopped
2 medium jars (6½ ounces *each*) marinated
 artichoke hearts, drained

1 bunch flat-leaf parsley, chopped
1 recipe Red Wine Vinaigrette (page 107)

Combine the hearts of palm, celery, artichoke hearts, and parsley in a salad bowl.

Toss with the vinaigrette. Season with salt and pepper and serve.

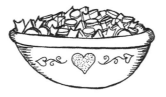

Crunchy Cabbage Salad

SERVES 6

Most coleslaws are made with carrots and mayonnaise dressings loaded with sugar. This is a tangy twist on classic coleslaw, perfect for backyard barbecues or picnics.

½ head green cabbage, shredded
½ head red cabbage, shredded
1 bunch parsley, chopped

1 medium red onion, thinly sliced
1 recipe Red Wine Vinaigrette (page 107)
Salt and freshly ground black pepper

Combine all the ingredients in a bowl. Refrigerate for at least an hour to let the flavors combine. Season with salt and pepper and serve.

Baby Artichoke Salad

SERVES 4

The baby artichokes used in this recipe are so tender that there is no need to cook them. Buy them fresh—don't use the marinated kind in a jar.

24 baby artichokes
6 lemons
5 tablespoons extra-virgin olive oil
¼ cup chopped flat-leaf parsley, plus
    4 sprigs for garnish

Salt and freshly ground black pepper
½ cup thin shavings of Parmesan cheese

Trim the bottoms and remove the tough outer green leaves from the baby artichokes until all that remains are the hearts with the yellowish tender leaves attached. Wash the trimmed artichokes and rub with the cut side of 1 lemon to prevent discoloration. Keep them in water with the juice from 1 lemon until ready to slice.

Slice the artichokes lengthwise *very thinly* (a mandolin is helpful). Toss with olive oil, the juice from 3 lemons, the parsley, salt, and pepper. Arrange on 4 plates and top with generous amounts of cheese shavings. Cut remaining lemon into quarters and garnish each plate with a lemon wedge and a sprig of parsley.

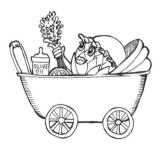

Cucumber Tomato Salad

PROTEINS/FATS AND VEGGIES; LEVEL ONE

SERVES 4

This crunchy little salad is a great starter.

2 medium cucumbers, seeded and chopped
4 medium tomatoes, chopped
1 medium red onion, thinly sliced

1 recipe Balsamic Vinaigrette (page 106)
Salt and freshly ground black pepper

Combine the cucumbers, tomatoes, and red onion in a medium bowl. Toss with the vinaigrette and season with salt and pepper.

Let marinate for about 30 minutes. (Do not refrigerate—the tomatoes will get mealy.)

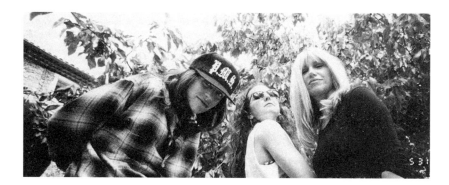

Leslie, Caroline, and me under
"Zee Famous Cherry Tree" in France.

Greek Salad

SERVES 4

This is always a winner and so simple to prepare. Makes you want to put a handkerchief between your teeth and dance.

3 medium tomatoes, chopped
1 medium cucumber, chopped
8 ounces feta cheese, crumbled
½ medium red onion, chopped
3 tablespoons extra-virgin olive oil

Juice from ½ lemon
Freshly ground black pepper
A pinch of dried oregano
Couple sprigs of fresh basil

Combine the tomatoes, cucumber, feta cheese, and red onion in a medium bowl. Mix, then drizzle with the olive oil and lemon juice. Grind the black pepper over the top of the salad, sprinkle with a touch of oregano, and garnish with basil sprigs. Adjust seasonings to taste.

For Level Two
Add Greek olives, if you like.

Chopped Salami and Vegetable Salad

PROTEINS/FATS AND VEGGIES: LEVEL ONE

SERVES 4

This is my version of the salad made so famous at the La Scala Boutique in Beverly Hills. It's another of Alan's favorite lunches. (He never realizes I am helping him keep his weight in check. He just likes my cooking.)

1 head iceberg lettuce, rinsed, dried, and
  chopped
¼ pound Italian dry salami, thinly sliced,
  then cut into thin strips
¼ pound mozzarella cheese, thinly sliced,
  then cut into thin strips

10 medium mushrooms, thinly sliced,
  then cut into thin strips
1 red bell pepper, stemmed, seeded, and
  julienned into thin strips
French Dressing (recipe follows)
8 whole peperoncini, for garnish

Combine the lettuce, salami, cheese, and vegetables in a bowl. Toss with dressing and arrange on 4 plates. Garnish with 2 peper-oncini on each salad. Season with additional salt and pepper.

French Dressing

MAKES ABOUT ¹/₂ CUP

Salt and freshly ground black pepper
1 teaspoon dry mustard
2 tablespoons tarragon vinegar
  (or white wine vinegar)

½ cup extra-virgin olive oil
1 teaspoon hot chili oil

Place the salt, pepper, mustard, and vine-gar in a small bowl and combine with a fork. Add the olive oil in a slow, steady stream, whisking constantly with a fork. Add the chili oil while continuing to whisk. Adjust seasonings to taste.

Grilled Chicken Salad with Sun-Dried Tomatoes and Goat Cheese

PROTEINS/FATS AND VEGGIES; LEVEL ONE

SERVES 4

I can eat this incredible salad—and lose weight. I serve this at luncheons, and my friends love it. The chicken can be pan-fried if you don't have a grill.

4 skinless and boneless chicken breasts
Salt and freshly ground black pepper
2 tablespoons olive oil
2 heads butter lettuce, leaves rinsed
  and dried

½ cup sun-dried tomatoes, drained and
  chopped
1 recipe Balsamic Vinaigrette (page 106)
10 ounces goat cheese, sliced into 8 rounds

Season the chicken breasts with salt and pepper. Cook over a hot grill, about 4 minutes per side, brushing with olive oil. Remove from heat and set aside.

Tear the lettuce into small pieces and toss with the sun-dried tomatoes and vinaigrette, reserving a few tablespoons to drizzle over the chicken and cheese. Arrange on 4 plates. Slice the chicken on the diagonal into ¼-inch-thick slices. Fan on top of the lettuce. Arrange 2 slices of goat cheese on each plate. Drizzle the remaining dressing over the chicken and cheese. Season with additional salt and pepper.

Grilled Chicken Salad with Watercress and Blue Cheese Vinaigrette

PROTEINS/FATS AND VEGGIES; LEVEL ONE

SERVES 4

I love blue cheese—and I can have it and still lose weight. The chicken in this salad can be pan-fried if you don't have a grill.

4 skinless and boneless chicken breasts
Salt and freshly ground black pepper
2 tablespoons olive oil
1 head red leaf lettuce, leaves rinsed
   and dried

2 bunches watercress, rinsed and dried
Blue Cheese Vinaigrette (recipe follows)
1 basket yellow cherry tomatoes, for
   garnish

Season the chicken breasts with salt and pepper. Cook over a hot grill, about 4 minutes per side, brushing with olive oil. Remove from the heat and set aside.

Tear the lettuce and watercress into small pieces and toss with the vinaigrette, reserving a few tablespoons to drizzle over the chicken. Arrange on 4 plates. Slice the chicken on the diagonal into ¼-inch-thick slices. Fan on top of the lettuce. Drizzle the remaining dressing over the chicken. Garnish with halved cherry tomatoes. Season with additional salt and pepper.

Blue Cheese Vinaigrette

MAKES ABOUT ³/4 CUP

6 ounces blue cheese (preferably a
   good Roquefort), crumbled

1 recipe Balsamic Vinaigrette
   (page 106)

Add the blue cheese to the vinaigrette and blend until combined.

Grilled Chicken Caesar Salad

PROTEINS/FATS AND VEGGIES; LEVEL ONE

SERVES 4

This is a favorite of mine—I don't eat anchovies, which are part of a classic Caesar salad, but you can add to the dressing four of the little buggers all mashed up if you really love them.

4 skinless and boneless chicken breasts
Salt and freshly ground black pepper
2 tablespoons olive oil
1 head romaine lettuce, rinsed and dried

Caesar Dressing (recipe follows)
1 lemon, quartered, for garnish

Season the chicken breasts with salt and pepper. Cook over a hot grill, about 4 minutes per side, brushing with olive oil. (Chicken can be pan-fried if you don't have a grill.) Remove from heat and set aside.

Tear the lettuce into small pieces and toss with dressing, reserving a few table-spoons to drizzle over the chicken. Arrange on 4 plates. Slice the chicken on the diagonal into ¼-inch-wide slices. Fan on top of the lettuce. Drizzle the remaining dressing over the chicken. Garnish with a lemon wedge. Season with additional salt and pepper.

Caesar Dressing

MAKES ABOUT ³/₄ CUP

1 egg
Juice from 1 lemon
Dash of Tabasco sauce

Salt and freshly ground black pepper
½ cup extra-virgin olive oil
½ cup freshly grated Parmesan cheese

Coddle the egg by boiling it in a saucepan for 20 seconds. Then remove the egg using a slotted spoon, crack it, and scoop out the inside into a medium bowl. Add the lemon juice, Tabasco, salt, and pepper to taste. Mix with a fork until well combined. Add the olive oil in a slow stream, stirring constantly. Finish by adding the cheese. Adjust seasonings to taste.

Tarragon Chicken Salad in Lettuce Cups

PROTEINS/FATS AND VEGGIES; LEVEL ONE

MAKES 4 TO 6 LETTUCE CUPS

I use lettuce leaves much as tortillas are used in Mexican food—I wrap fillings in them. Many people say this tastes better than a traditional bread sandwich.

CHICKEN SALAD

2 cups chopped cooked chicken

3 tablespoons Homemade Mayonnaise
(page 86)

3 celery stalks, finely chopped

¼ sweet onion (Maui or Vidalia), finely
chopped

½ red bell pepper, finely chopped

2 tablespoons chopped fresh tarragon
(or ½ teaspoon dried)

Salt and freshly ground black pepper

LETTUCE CUPS

4 to 6 romaine lettuce leaves

3 green onions, chopped

Sprigs of fresh tarragon, for garnish

Place all ingredients for chicken salad in a bowl and mix until well combined. Adjust seasonings.

Place a large dollop of chicken salad in each lettuce leaf. Garnish with green onions and tarragon. Then fold it up like a taco and enjoy.

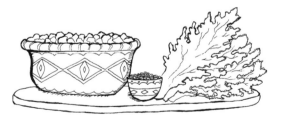

Tuna Salad in Lettuce Cups

PROTEINS/FATS AND VEGGIES; LEVEL ONE

MAKES 4 TO 6 LETTUCE CUPS

There are so many ways to use lettuce leaves in place of bread. This is my version of a tuna salad sandwich.

TUNA SALAD

1 can (12 ounces) tuna, drained (I like
    white albacore packed in water)
4 tablespoons Homemade Mayonnaise
    (page 86)
3 celery stalks, finely chopped
½ medium red onion, finely chopped
Juice from 1 lemon

Place ingredients for tuna salad in a bowl and mix until well combined. Adjust seasonings.

Freshly ground black pepper
½ teaspoon dried dill

LETTUCE CUPS

4 to 6 iceberg lettuce leaves
2 to 3 plum tomatoes, chopped
3 green onions, chopped

Place a large dollop of tuna salad in each lettuce leaf, garnish with tomatoes and green onions. Fold it up like a taco and enjoy.

Salmon Salad with Watercress in Lettuce Cups

PROTEINS/FATS AND VEGGIES; LEVEL ONE

MAKES 4 TO 6 LETTUCE CUPS

SALMON SALAD

1 can (12 ounces) or steamed fresh salmon, drained
4 tablespoons Homemade Mayonnaise (page 86)
½ cup coarsely chopped watercress
½ medium cucumber, peeled, seeded, and finely chopped

Juice from 1 lemon
Freshly ground black pepper

LETTUCE CUPS

4 to 6 radicchio leaves
2 to 3 medium tomatoes, chopped
Chopped watercress, for garnish

Place ingredients for salmon salad in a bowl and mix until well combined. Adjust seasonings.

Place a large dollop of salmon salad in each radicchio leaf, garnish with tomatoes and a little extra watercress. Fold it up like a taco and enjoy.

Egg Salad in Lettuce Cups

PROTEINS/FATS AND VEGGIES; LEVEL ONE

MAKES 4 TO 6 LETTUCE CUPS

EGG SALAD

8 eggs
4 tablespoons Homemade Mayonnaise
   (page 86)
3 celery stalks, finely chopped
10 chives *or* 5 green onions, finely chopped
Salt and freshly ground black pepper

LETTUCE CUPS

4 to 6 butter lettuce leaves
Handful of onion sprouts (optional)
Chives, for garnish

Place the eggs in a pan filled with enough cold water to cover them. Bring the water to a boil, then lower the heat to medium and cook for 15 minutes. Drain the hot water and run the hard-boiled eggs under cold water until cool enough to peel. Dice the peeled eggs and place in a bowl.

Add the remaining salad ingredients, adjusting the seasonings.

Place a large dollop of egg salad in each lettuce leaf, garnish with a few onion sprouts, if desired, and additional chives. Fold it up like a taco and enjoy.

Taco Salad

SERVES 4

If you like Mexican food, you'll love this hearty taco salad!

2 tablespoons vegetable oil
1 medium onion, chopped
5 garlic cloves, pressed
1 pound ground beef
1 teaspoon paprika
1 teaspoon ground cumin
½ teaspoon dried oregano
½ teaspoon chili powder
½ teaspoon cayenne
Salt and freshly ground black pepper

1 cup water
1 can (6 ounces) tomato paste
1 head romaine lettuce, leaves rinsed, dried, and chopped
2 medium tomatoes, chopped
6 ounces Cheddar cheese, grated
6 tablespoons sour cream
6 green onions, chopped
1 jar (8 ounces) Mexican salsa

In a large skillet over medium heat, heat the oil. Add the onion and cook until translucent, about 4 minutes. Add the garlic and cook for 1 minute longer. Turn up the heat to high and add the ground beef. Brown the meat, stirring constantly, until crumbly, about 4 minutes. Drain excess fat. Lower heat and add the paprika, cumin, oregano, chili powder, cayenne, and plenty of salt and pepper. Add the water and tomato paste, blending well with a wooden spoon. Bring to a boil, then reduce the heat to low and simmer for 10 minutes, stirring occasionally.

To assemble the salad, place the romaine on 4 plates. Spoon the meat mixture over the lettuce. Top with tomatoes, cheese, sour cream, green onions, and salsa.

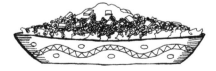

Soups and Sandwiches

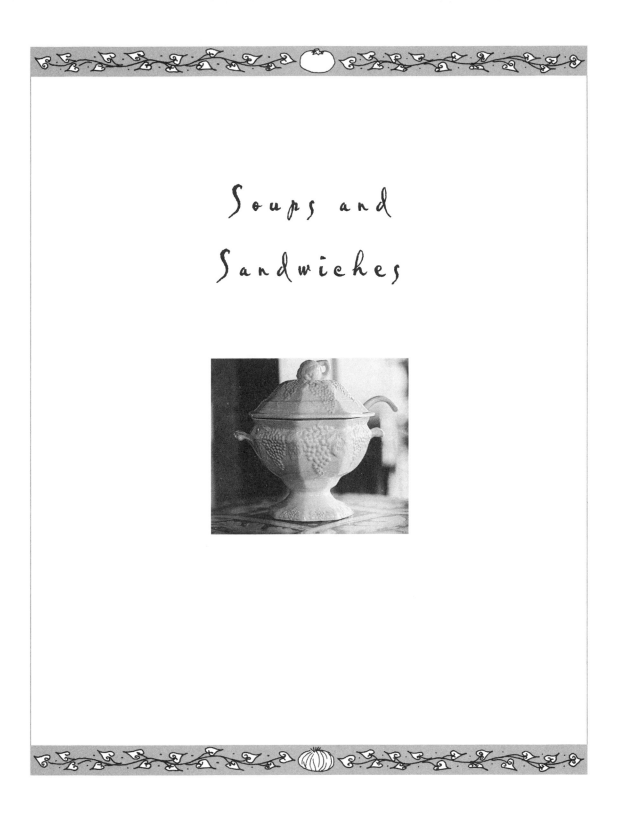

Grandma's Traditional Chicken Soup

PROTEINS/FATS AND VEGGIES; LEVEL ONE

SERVES 6

When you're feeling blue or out of sorts, this is the world's best medicine. And when you're feeling good, this is the best chicken soup to serve on a cold winter night. It's great with a sprinkle of Parmesan cheese or a dollop of pesto on top.

BROTH

1 chicken (3 pounds) or meaty chicken
  carcass
1 medium onion, halved
3 celery stalks, roughly chopped
3 parsnips, roughly chopped
Stems from 1 bunch parsley
A handful (approximately 25) whole black
  peppercorns

SOUP

5 celery stalks, chopped
5 parsnips, peeled and chopped
3 leeks, cleaned well and chopped
1 bunch parsley, chopped
Salt and freshly ground black pepper

For the broth: Place the chicken or chicken carcass into a large stockpot. Fill with water to cover. Add the remaining stock ingredients and cook over very low heat for 8 to 10 hours. Strain the broth, discarding the vegetables but reserving the carcass. Place the broth into a container and refrigerate. When the broth is chilled, skim off the fat that has risen to the top.

Pick the meat off the chicken or carcass, being careful to remove any bones, skin, fat, and tendons. (This is a tedious process, but well worth the effort.) Reserve the meat and discard the bones.

For the soup: Reheat the defatted chicken broth in a stockpot. Add the celery, parsnips, leeks, parsley, and chicken meat. Cook until vegetables are tender, about 20 minutes over medium heat. Season with salt and pepper.

For Level Two
Add 1 cup cooked wild rice.

Incredible Chicken Broth

PROTEINS/FATS AND VEGGIES; LEVEL ONE

MAKES 2 QUARTS (ENOUGH FOR 8 PEOPLE)

Every good cook has fresh chicken stock available to make the best-tasting soups and sauces. My friend Paula Marshall gave me this recipe many years ago, and it's a winner! I like to keep it in small airtight containers in the freezer, so I can quickly defrost it as needed for sauces and quick soups.

5 pounds chicken wings
1 head garlic, unpeeled
2 leeks, washed and cut into thirds
5 shallots, peeled
8 celery stalks (including leaves), cut
    into thirds

Salt to taste
20 black peppercorns
3 sprigs fresh thyme
1 bunch parsley

Place all the ingredients in a stockpot and add water to cover. Bring to a boil, then turn down to lowest heat. Cover and simmer on the lowest possible setting for about 3 hours.

Strain the broth and discard all other ingredients. Put broth in the refrigerator and let fat harden on top, about 4 hours. Skim fat off the top when cooled, and discard.

Chicken Tomato Cilantro Soup

PROTEINS/FATS AND VEGGIES; LEVEL ONE

SERVES 6

Make this soup from the leftovers of my Roasted Herbes de Provence Chicken (page 164). If you start the soup while you're cleaning up, you'll have dinner the next night without really trying.

Cooked chicken carcass and any veggies,
   sauce, and juices from roasting pan
Salt and freshly ground black pepper
1 can (28 ounces) Italian plum tomatoes,
   with juice

1 teaspoon dried oregano
6 tablespoons chopped fresh cilantro

Remove any leftover meat from the carcass and set aside. Put the carcass in a soup pot and cover with water. Add any leftover vegetables and sauce, then salt and pepper to taste. Heat to a boil, then lower heat and simmer for about 3 hours.

Strain the broth, discarding the bones and vegetables. Refrigerate broth until the fat hardens on top, about 4 hours. Skim off the fat and return broth to the stove to reheat over medium heat.

Roughly chop the tomatoes and add them to the broth with their juice. Then add the oregano, leftover chicken, and additional salt and pepper to taste. Cook over medium heat for 30 minutes, then serve the soup hot, with a sprinkle of cilantro.

"Tom Yum Kai" Spicy Thai Chicken Soup

PROTEINS/FATS AND VEGGIES; LEVEL ONE

SERVES 6

If you're feeling adventurous, this traditional Thai chicken soup is spicy and delicious. Some of the ingredients can be hard to find, but the result is well worth the effort if you succeed. There is a Bangkok market in Los Angeles where I get most of the ingredients. The lemongrass, lime leaves, chilies, ginger, and galangal are not to be eaten; they are added only for flavor.

2 quarts chicken broth
3 stalks lemongrass, cut into large pieces
¼ cup kaffir lime leaves
2 to 5 serrano chilies
¼ cup Thai fish sauce
12 slices peeled ginger
6 slices peeled galangal

2 skinless and boneless chicken breasts,
    cut into bite-size pieces
12 cherry tomatoes, halved
½ cup coarsely chopped cilantro
1 can (16 ounces) straw mushrooms,
    drained
Juice from 2 limes

Heat the chicken broth in a large stock-pot. Add the lemongrass, lime leaves, chilies, fish sauce, ginger, and galangal. Lower the heat and simmer for 30 minutes or more. (At this point you can strain the broth, if you like. I prefer to keep all of the items in for extra flavor and a more beautiful presentation.)

Add the chicken, cherry tomatoes, cilantro, straw mushrooms, and lime juice. Simmer an additional 30 minutes, then serve.

Oriental Turkey Meatball Soup

PROTEINS/FATS AND VEGGIES; LEVEL ONE

SERVES 4

This recipe is best when made with fresh chicken broth (any of the broths in this book would be wonderful). For those rare occasions when I'm out of fresh, I like to keep a case of canned chicken broth in my pantry. I use it for flavoring sauces and for quick soups, like this one.

6 cups chicken broth (page 125)
1 pound ground turkey, rolled into
   1-inch balls
2 celery stalks, finely chopped

5 slices fresh ginger, peeled
2 tablespoons soy sauce
½ teaspoon hot chili oil
2 heads baby bok choy

Bring the broth to a boil and add the turkey balls, celery, ginger, soy sauce, and chili oil. Reduce the heat and simmer for 30 minutes. Then add the bok choy and simmer for an additional 5 minutes. Adjust the flavor with additional soy sauce and chili oil. Serve immediately.

Mushroom Lemon Soup

PROTEINS/FATS AND VEGGIES; LEVEL ONE

SERVES 6

My neighbor Diane gave me this recipe. It's easy and delicious. Fresh shiitake mushrooms or any other kind of wild mushroom make the soup fantastic, but white mushrooms also work and are quite delicious. This is great with hot Whole Wheat Popovers (page 193).

2 onions, quartered
1 pound shiitake mushrooms
3 tablespoons olive oil

6 cups chicken broth (page 125)
Salt and freshly ground black pepper
4 lemons, 3 halved and 1 sliced thin

Puree the onions in a food processor.

Clean the mushrooms by gently dusting with a mushroom brush, then finely chop in a food processor.

In a medium saucepan, heat the olive oil. Cook the onions in the saucepan until transparent. Then add the mushrooms and cook for 4 minutes. Add the chicken broth, salt, and pepper, and simmer for 30 minutes.

Ladle the soup into bowls and squeeze the juice from ½ lemon into each bowl. Garnish each bowl with a lemon slice.

Lentil Soup

SERVES 10 TO 12

Lentils are known to cause gas, which is why I've added the fresh ginger. According to my mother, it takes away the gas. I don't know why, but it works! It tastes good, too.

1 pound lentils
6 cups Vegetable Broth (page 132) or water
2 slices of fresh ginger
1 medium onion, chopped
Salt and freshly ground black pepper

2 bunches cilantro, stemmed and chopped
5 lemons
1 bunch basil, stemmed and chopped
Lemon slices, for garnish

Place the lentils in a stockpot. Add the broth, ginger, and onion. Bring to a boil, reduce the heat, and simmer for about 90 minutes, or until the lentils are tender.

Transfer the lentil mixture to a blender or food processor and blend for 30 seconds.

Add the salt, pepper, and cilantro.

Ladle the soup into bowls and squeeze the juice of 1/2 lemon into each bowl. Garnish with liberal amounts of the basil and a thin slice of lemon.

Roasted Red Pepper Soup

SERVES 6

This vegetarian soup features flavorful red bell peppers. Because it's made only with vegetables, it can be eaten with either Carbos or Proteins/Fats.

3 cups Vegetable Broth (page 132)
12 Roasted Red Peppers (page 81)
1 medium red onion, chopped

2 garlic cloves
¼ teaspoon hot red pepper flakes
Salt and freshly ground black pepper

In a stockpot, bring the Vegetable Broth to a boil. Add the red peppers, onion, garlic, and red pepper flakes. Bring back to a boil, then immediately reduce the heat and simmer for about 10 minutes.

Transfer to a blender or food processor and blend until smooth. Add salt and pepper to taste.

For a Carbos and Veggies Meal
Garnish with nonfat yogurt and freshly chopped cilantro. Serve with toasted whole-grain bread.

For a Proteins/Fats and Veggies Meal
Garnish with sour cream and freshly chopped cilantro. Serve with a grilled chicken breast and a green salad. (You may prepare the soup with Chicken Broth, page 125, for additional flavor.)

Vegetable Broth

MAKES ABOUT 8 CUPS

6 quarts water
2 heads garlic, unpeeled
4 medium onions, halved
5 parsnips, roughly chopped
5 leeks, washed and roughly chopped

1 bunch parsley
1 bunch thyme
5 bay leaves
5 celery stalks
25 whole black peppercorns

In a large stockpot, combine all the ingredients and bring to a boil. Reduce heat and simmer for 3 hours. Strain and discard the vegetables and peppercorns.

Note If you're using this broth with Proteins/Fats, it tastes even better if you first sauté the vegetables in olive oil before adding the water.

Broccoli Leek Soup

PROTEINS/FATS AND VEGGIES; LEVEL ONE

SERVES 6

A nice light supper—wonderful on Level Two with hot Whole Wheat Popovers (page 193). A tasty soup you will enjoy year-round. The fried leeks and garlic sprinkled on top of the soup add to the flavor.

¼ cup olive oil
2 leeks, trimmed of dark green leaves,
    then cleaned and chopped
8 cups chicken broth
6 cups (about 3 stalks) chopped broccoli
    florets
Salt and freshly ground black pepper

FRIED LEEKS

6 tablespoons olive oil
1 leek, trimmed of dark green leaves, then
    cleaned and very thinly sliced
3 garlic cloves, finely chopped

6 tablespoons sour cream

Heat the olive oil in a large stockpot. Add the leeks and sauté for about 5 minutes, until they are lightly browned. Add the chicken broth and bring to a boil. Add the broccoli and bring back to a boil, then immediately reduce the heat and simmer for 15 minutes, until broccoli is soft. Season with salt and pepper. Transfer to a blender or food processor and blend until smooth.

For the fried leeks: Heat the olive oil in a skillet over medium heat, then add half the leeks and cook until golden brown. Remove with a slotted spoon and drain on paper towels. Repeat these steps with the remaining leeks. Finally, fry the garlic until golden brown. Set aside with the leeks.

Ladle the soup into individual bowls and garnish each with a dollop of sour cream. Top with the fried leeks and garlic.

Cold Cucumber Asparagus Soup

CARBOS AND VEGGIES; LEVEL ONE

SERVES 4

This is a beautiful, vibrant, green, light summer soup. It has no added fat, which makes it a perfect starter for a Carbos and Veggies meal.

1½ cups chopped asparagus (about 35 stalks), tough ends removed
2 cups Vegetable Broth (page 132)
2 medium cucumbers, peeled, seeded, and chopped
1 tablespoon finely chopped fresh dill
Salt and freshly ground black pepper

GARNISH

4 tablespoons plain nonfat yogurt
4 sprigs fresh dill

Place about 2 cups of water in the bottom of a pan fitted with a steaming basket and a lid. Heat on high until the water boils. Put the asparagus in the steamer, cover, and cook until tender, approximately 4 minutes. Remove the asparagus and rinse under cool water. Transfer the cooled asparagus to a blender or food processor. Add the Vegetable Broth, cucumbers, and dill. Blend until smooth.

Season the soup with salt and pepper. Chill in the refrigerator at least 1 hour, then serve with dollops of nonfat yogurt and garnished with a sprig of fresh dill.

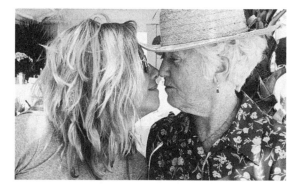

I have the best mom.

Pita Sandwiches with Veggies and Yogurt Cheese

CARBOS AND VEGGIES; LEVEL ONE

SERVES 2

These sandwiches can be made with any of your favorite vegetables. Instead of the yogurt cheese, try Baba Ganoush (page 75) or Hummus (page 77).

2 whole wheat pitas
4 Roasted Red Peppers (page 81,
    or jarred roasted peppers)
2 slices sweet onion
½ medium cucumber, thinly sliced

A few arugula leaves (or red leaf lettuce)
Yogurt Cheese (recipe follows)
Drizzle of balsamic vinegar
¼ teaspoon dried oregano
Salt and freshly ground black pepper

Slice one edge off the pita breads to make a pouch with an opening. Toast the pita, then fill with the peppers, onion, cucumber, and arugula.

Spoon some of the Yogurt Cheese on the vegetables and drizzle balsamic vinegar over it. Then sprinkle with oregano, salt, and pepper.

Yogurt Cheese

MAKES ENOUGH CHEESE FOR 4 SANDWICHES

1 cup plain nonfat yogurt

Line a fine strainer with cheesecloth. Place the yogurt in the strainer with a bowl underneath to catch the liquid. Refrigerate overnight. Most of the moisture will drain out of the yogurt, creating a soft, delicious cheese.

Use a portion of the cheese for the sandwiches and refrigerate the rest to eat later.

Chicken and Roasted Vegetable Sandwiches

PROTEINS/FATS AND VEGGIES; LEVEL ONE

MAKES 4 SANDWICHES

The vegetables serve as the bread in these delicious little chicken sandwiches. You can see how beautiful they look in the poolside picture on the back cover of this book.

ROASTED VEGETABLES

1 large eggplant, cut lengthwise into
   8 slices, about ⅓ inch thick
Caps of 8 large shiitake mushrooms
3 medium zucchini, cut lengthwise into
   ¼-inch slices
2 medium red onions, cut into ¼-inch slices
8 ripe medium tomatoes, sliced in half
   crosswise
2 to 3 tablespoons olive oil
2 teaspoons balsamic vinegar
½ teaspoon chopped fresh thyme leaves

Salt and freshly ground black pepper
¼ teaspoon hot red pepper flakes

CHICKEN BREASTS

2 skinless and boneless chicken breasts,
   separated into halves
2 teaspoons dried rosemary
Salt and freshly ground black pepper
2 tablespoons olive oil
½ pound fresh mozzarella cheese, cut
   into ¼-inch slices
Sprigs of fresh rosemary (optional)

Preheat the oven to 425° F.

For the vegetables: Place the eggplant, mushrooms, zucchini, onions, and tomatoes on baking sheets. In a small bowl, combine the olive oil, vinegar, thyme, salt, pepper, and red pepper flakes. Lightly brush on the vegetables and bake, removing the vegetables as they each become golden brown (the zucchini and eggplant in about 15 minutes, then the mushrooms and onions; the tomatoes will take up to 45 minutes).

For the chicken breasts: Place each breast between pieces of plastic wrap and pound with a mallet until about ⅓ inch thick. Season with rosemary, salt, and pepper. Heat a large skillet over medium-high heat. Add a little olive oil and sauté the chicken on each side until nicely browned and just cooked through, about 5 minutes.

Assemble the sandwiches on a baking sheet, using the eggplant as the "bread." On a slice of eggplant, layer a chicken piece, then mozzarella, tomato, zucchini, 2 mushrooms, and onion, ending with another eggplant slice. (You may have to trim the chicken and zucchini to fit the shape of the eggplant slices.) Secure the sandwiches with toothpicks or sprigs of rosemary. Heat on baking sheet for another 5 minutes or until the mozzarella has melted.

Meatless
Main Dishes

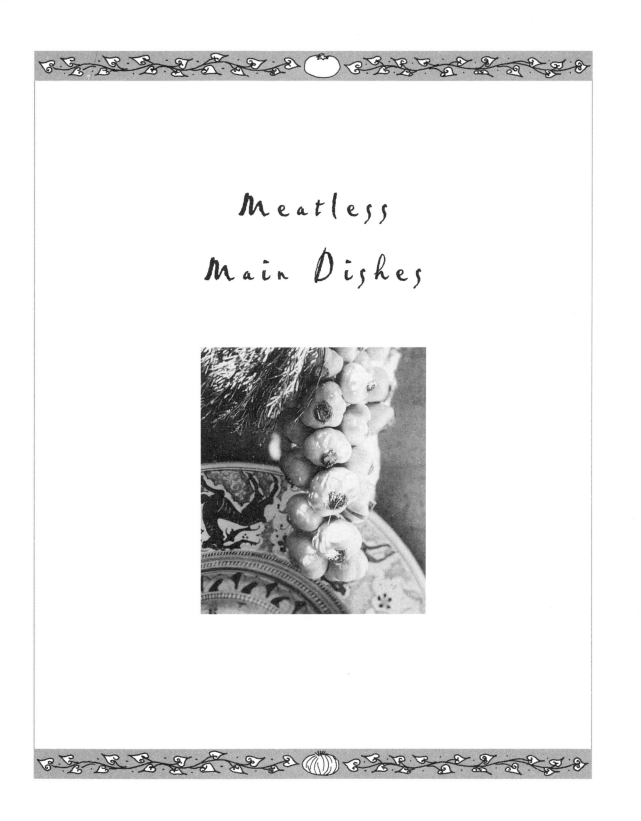

Flourless Cheese Soufflé

PROTEINS/FATS; LEVEL ONE

SERVES 4

This tastes too good to be true, but it is. I like it as a Saturday lunch, when we're hanging around the house, listening to classical music.

2 tablespoons butter, softened
6 large eggs, separated
Pinch of cayenne pepper
½ teaspoon freshly grated nutmeg

Salt and freshly ground black pepper
4 ounces cream cheese, softened
1½ cups finely grated Gruyère or
   Swiss cheese

Preheat the oven to 425°F. Coat a 6-cup soufflé dish with the butter.

In a mixing bowl, combine the egg yolks, cayenne, nutmeg, salt, and pepper. Beat with a wire whisk until light and fluffy. Add the cream cheese and grated cheese and whisk until well combined and smooth.

In another bowl, beat the egg whites until somewhat stiff peaks form. Fold the egg whites into the cheese mixture. Spoon into the greased dish and place on a baking sheet.

Bake for 10 minutes. Reduce the heat to 400°F and bake an additional 15 minutes. Serve immediately.

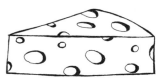

Zucchini Frittata

SERVES 2

A light and easy breakfast, lunch, or dinner. For dinner, I often serve this with a simple green salad.

4 large eggs
Salt and freshly ground black pepper
2 tablespoons olive oil
1 medium onion, chopped

½ cup julienned zucchini
Sprinkle of grated Parmesan cheese
1 medium tomato, seeded and diced
10 fresh basil leaves, chopped

Preheat the oven to 350° F.

Whisk the eggs in a bowl with a splash of water. Add a dash of salt and pepper. Place a medium sauté pan (with an ovenproof handle) over medium heat. When the pan is hot, add the olive oil. Sauté the onion until crispy brown, about 10 minutes, then set aside half the onion for a garnish. Add the zucchini to the remaining onion in the hot pan and sauté for a few minutes.

Add the beaten eggs to the sauté pan.

Immediately sprinkle with the grated cheese and remove from the heat.

Place the pan in the preheated oven. (If you do not have a sauté pan with an ovenproof handle, transfer the egg mixture at this point to a small casserole dish or pie pan.) Bake for 7 to 10 minutes, until puffy and golden.

While the frittata is baking, in a separate bowl mix the tomato, basil, and salt and pepper to taste. Top the cooked frittata with the tomato mixture and garnish with crispy onions.

Zucchini Pancakes with Warm Tomato Coulis

PROTEINS/FATS AND VEGGIES; LEVEL ONE

SERVES 6

I love these pancakes for brunch or lunch. They taste best when served hot right out of the pan, but you can also make them in advance and serve them at room temperature.

TOMATO COULIS

3 tablespoons olive oil
1 medium onion, diced
2 garlic cloves, minced
3 large, ripe tomatoes, peeled, seeded, and
    diced (or 6 canned Italian plum
    tomatoes, seeded)
5 bay leaves
1 teaspoon chopped fresh thyme
Salt and freshly ground black pepper

ZUCCHINI PANCAKES

1 large zucchini, shredded
3 large eggs
3 tablespoons chopped parsley
¾ teaspoon salt
½ teaspoon ground white pepper
2 tablespoons unsalted butter

Grated fresh Parmesan cheese, for garnish

For the coulis: Heat the oil in a medium skillet over moderate heat. Sauté the onion until golden brown, about 15 minutes. Add the garlic and sauté for 1 more minute. Add the tomatoes, bay leaves, thyme, salt, and pepper. Reduce to a simmer and cook uncovered for 15 minutes. Remove the bay leaves. Keep warm.

For the pancakes: Preheat the broiler. In a bowl, mix the zucchini with the eggs, parsley, salt, and pepper.

Melt 1 tablespoon of the butter in a small nonstick ovenproof skillet over medium-high heat. (I usually get 2 skillets going at the same time, one for each pancake. If you don't have 2 skillets, keep the first pancake in a warm oven while you make the second.) Add half of the zucchini mixture and reduce heat to low. Gently cook for 3 to 5 minutes, shaking the pan occasionally. The pancake should be loose in the center but set around the edges. Transfer the skillet to the broiler. Cook until firm in the center, about 4 minutes. (If you don't have a skillet with an ovenproof handle, you can flip the pancake by inverting it onto a plate, browned side up. Then slide it back into the skillet to cook the other side.) Repeat for second pancake.

Slice each pancake into 3 wedges and center on serving plates. Garnish with tomato coulis and sprinkle with Parmesan cheese. Serve immediately.

Ricotta Pancake

SERVES 2

This is good for a light lunch or supper with a green salad. It's great with my Simple Tomato, Basil, and Garlic Sauce (page 145).

1½ cups ricotta cheese
4 large eggs
1 teaspoon fennel seeds

Salt and freshly ground black pepper
1 tablespoon olive oil

Place the ricotta in a medium bowl and add the eggs, one at a time, stirring well after each addition. Add the fennel, salt, and pepper.

Heat the olive oil briefly in a large skillet over medium heat. Pour in the egg-ricotta mixture to make one large pancake. Gently move the mixture around with a wooden spoon until the egg sets, about 5 to 6 minutes. The surface will still be a little runny. Invert the pancake onto a plate, cooked side up. Then slide the pancake back into the skillet to cook the other side for 1 to 2 minutes more. Slice into 6 wedges and serve immediately.

Whole Wheat Cheeseless Pizza

CARBOS AND VEGGIES; LEVEL ONE

SERVES 4

These individual pizzas are incredibly easy to prepare. Top with your favorite vegetables. You can even melt some fat-free mozzarella cheese on the veggies, if you like.

4 whole wheat pitas
1 cup Simple Tomato, Basil, and Garlic
   Sauce (page 145)
1 medium tomato, thinly sliced
½ cup thinly sliced mushrooms

½ medium onion, thinly sliced
12 artichoke hearts (fresh or packed
   in water, not oil)

Preheat the oven to 425°F.

Place the pitas on a baking sheet. Spread the tomato sauce evenly over the pitas. Arrange the tomato slices over the sauce, then sprinkle on the mushrooms, onion, and artichoke hearts. Cook for 15 to 20 minutes, or until bubbly.

For Level Two
Top with a little Parmesan cheese.

Black Bean Chili with Spicy Tomato Salsa

CARBOS AND VEGGIES; LEVEL ONE

SERVES 6

Serve with lavash bread or a fat-free whole wheat tortilla. This is yummy and contains no added fat! Use leftover chili the next day spooned inside a warmed whole wheat tortilla with salsa to make a black bean burrito.

BLACK BEAN CHILI

1 pound dried black beans, soaked overnight and drained, or fresh black beans (they can be used immediately)
1 medium onion, diced
3 garlic cloves, minced
4 serrano chilies, finely chopped
Salt and freshly ground black pepper

For the chili: Place the beans in a large stockpot. Add water until the level is 2 inches above the beans. Add the onion, garlic, and chilies. Turn the heat to high. As the beans heat up, skim the foam off the top. When the beans come to a boil, turn the heat to low and simmer until tender,

SPICY TOMATO SALSA

4 medium tomatoes, diced
½ medium cucumber, diced
1 bunch cilantro, coarsely chopped
1 medium red onion, diced
2 serrano chilies, finely chopped
1 garlic clove, minced
Juice from 2 limes

about 1 hour. Season with salt and pepper.

For the salsa: Gently combine all the salsa ingredients in a nonreactive bowl and set aside for the flavors to combine, about 30 minutes.

Serve chili in bowls with a large spoonful of salsa.

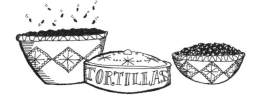

Roasted Vegetable Lasagne

CARBOS AND VEGGIES; LEVEL ONE

SERVES 6

Lasagne is a lot of work, so it better be worth it. This one is. And of course, the great thing with lasagne is that it can be made a day in advance. It actually tastes better *that way because the flavors have time to meld.*

4 medium zucchini, sliced lengthwise
    into ⅛-inch slices
1 large eggplant, sliced lengthwise
    into ⅛-inch slices
20 medium tomatoes, cut in half crosswise
Salt and freshly ground black pepper
3 tablespoons chopped fresh thyme

2 cups nonfat ricotta cheese
1 head Baked Garlic (page 80)
1 pound spinach or whole-grain lasagne
    noodles
1 recipe Simple Tomato, Basil, and Garlic
    Sauce (opposite)
8 Roasted Red Peppers (see page 81)

Preheat the oven to 425°F.

Lay the zucchini, eggplant, and tomatoes cut side up on baking sheets. Sprinkle with salt, pepper, and 1 tablespoon of thyme. Roast until golden brown. The zucchini and eggplant will take about 15 minutes, the tomatoes about 45 minutes. Lower the oven temperature to 350°F.

Combine the ricotta, garlic, remaining thyme, and salt and pepper in a bowl.

Cook the pasta according to package instructions. Rinse with cool water, then lay the pieces out flat so they don't stick together.

To assemble the lasagne, pour a thin layer of tomato sauce (½ cup) on the bottom of a 13 x 9-inch pan. Lay 3 lasagne noodles lengthwise in the pan. Then add half of the ricotta and garlic mixture, a layer of roasted peppers, and a layer of zucchini, then another layer of pasta, the rest of the cheese mixture, another ½ cup of sauce, then the eggplant and tomatoes. Top with a layer of pasta, ending with more tomato sauce.

Cover with foil and bake about 45 minutes or until bubbling. Remove from the oven and let stand for 10 minutes before serving.

Penne with Simple Tomato, Basil, and Garlic Sauce

CARBOS AND VEGGIES; LEVEL ONE

SERVES 6

I always keep these ingredients stocked so I can whip up this meal in just minutes. It's fast, simple, and delicious!

SAUCE

2 cans (28 ounces each) peeled tomatoes, coarsely chopped with juice
1 medium onion, chopped
6 garlic cloves, sliced very thin

Salt and freshly ground black pepper
20 fresh basil leaves, stacked, rolled, and sliced thin

1 pound whole-grain penne pasta

Over medium-high heat, warm about ⅓ cup of the juice from the peeled tomatoes in a saucepan. Add the onion and sauté until soft, about 7 minutes. Then add the garlic and sauté another 3 minutes. (If the tomato juice is bubbling too much, turn the heat down to medium.) Add the remaining tomatoes and their juice. Lower the heat and simmer for 20 minutes. Add salt and pepper. Stir and cook for an additional 5 minutes. Turn off the heat and add the basil.

Cook the pasta according to package instructions. Toss with the sauce and serve immediately.

For Level Two
Start the sauce by sautéing the onion for about 10 minutes (until golden brown) in about ½ cup extra-virgin olive oil. Add the garlic and cook until just pale gold. Turn down the heat and add the tomatoes with their juice. Finish as above. The oil adds a delicious flavor and helps release the sweetness of the onion and the garlic. This addition creates only a small imbalance, which is fine for Level Two. If you want to add Parmesan cheese, your imbalance goes up another notch.

Whole Wheat Artichoke Pasta with Fresh Tomato Sauce

CARBOS AND VEGGIES; LEVEL ONE

SERVES 4

This is the sauce Italian women traditionally make when tomatoes are in season. It has an amazingly pure, fresh taste. Make it when you have fresh tomatoes that are so wonderful they will stand on their own. This is a great sauce by itself, but you can also add fresh veggies, including onions, garlic, peppers, and mushrooms. Just remember—no Proteins/Fats in this Level One Carbos meal.

SAUCE

12 to 15 vine-ripened tomatoes, halved crosswise
Salt and freshly ground black pepper
½ teaspoon hot red pepper flakes

1 pound whole wheat Jerusalem artichoke pasta (or other whole-grain pasta)
A few sprigs of Italian flat-leaf parsley

Place the tomatoes, cut side up, in a large saucepan. Cover with a fitted lid. Cook over very low heat for approximately 40 minutes. Gently mash the tomatoes and add salt, pepper, and red pepper flakes to taste.

Cook the pasta according to package instructions. Drain the pasta and place on a large platter. Cover with the fresh tomato sauce and garnish with the parsley.

For Level Two
You can add a little Parmesan cheese or add vegetables sautéed in a little olive oil, such as onions, garlic, peppers, and mushrooms.

Fish and Seafood

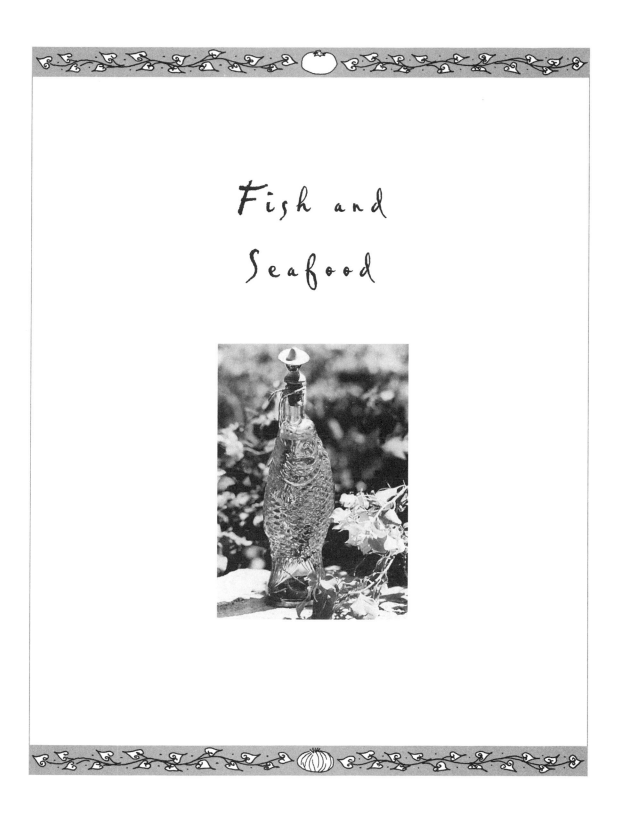

Citrus-Marinated Barbecued Shrimp with Fresh Arugula

PROTEINS/FATS AND VEGGIES; LEVEL ONE

SERVES 4

This is tangy and spicy. Makes you want to do the cha-cha!

SHRIMP

20 large shrimp, peeled and deveined
7 garlic cloves, pressed
1 bunch cilantro, chopped
½ cup olive oil
3 serrano chilies, chopped
Zest from 1 lime
Juice from 3 limes

ARUGULA

1 pound fresh arugula, rinsed and dried
2 teaspoons olive oil
Juice from 1 lemon
Salt and freshly ground black pepper

For the shrimp: Combine all the ingredients in a noncorrosive bowl. Marinate the shrimp for 30 minutes. Prepare the grill. Cook the shrimp over a hot grill, basting with the marinade until just cooked through. Do not overcook the shrimp, or they will get tough. Keep warm.

For the arugula: Toss the arugula with olive oil, lemon juice, and salt and pepper.

Arrange on 4 plates. To serve, position the shrimp in a lovely pattern on top of the arugula.

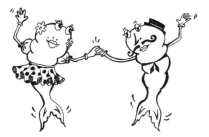

Salmon Steaks with Fried Ginger and Lime

PROTEINS/FATS AND VEGGIES; LEVEL ONE

SERVES 4

Great with steamed asparagus! This salmon is topped with yummy little fried pieces of ginger and fresh crispy vegetables that have an Asian flair.

FRIED GINGER

1 piece (3 inches long) fresh ginger
½ cup vegetable oil

SALMON

4 salmon steaks
2 tablespoons olive oil

Salt and freshly ground black pepper
1 lime, sliced paper thin with peel
2 Kirby cucumbers, halved lengthwise
    and sliced thin
A handful of daikon sprouts (optional)
3 tablespoons soy sauce
Juice from 1 lime

For the ginger: Peel the ginger and thinly slice. Cut the slices into thin strips. Heat the vegetable oil in a frying pan. When hot, add the ginger and cook until dark golden brown. Remove with a slotted spoon; set aside to drain on paper towels.

For the salmon: Prepare the grill. Brush the salmon with a little olive oil, then season with salt and pepper. Cook on a hot grill until just cooked through; cooking time will vary depending on the thickness of the fish, from 5 to 15 minutes.

Cut each lime slice into 8 pieces, as if you were cutting a pie. Toss the lime with the cucumbers and daikon sprouts in a mixture of the soy sauce and lime juice. Place the salmon on 4 individual plates and heap the vegetable garnish on the fish. Top with a sprinkle of fried ginger.

Braised Salmon in White Wine and Fresh Ginger

PROTEINS/FATS AND VEGGIES; LEVEL ONE

SERVES 12

Along with his wife, my dear friend and Step by Step *costar Patrick Duffy made this for Alan and me at their beloved Oregon home. The fish was pulled from the river, and two hours later the four of us were licking our lips over it. This recipe is easy and incredibly delicious. You don't have to use whole salmon; salmon steaks or fillets will work just fine. (Just be sure to drastically adjust the cooking time.)*

1 bottle chardonnay
   (or any other dry white wine)
2 lemons
⅓ cup peeled and grated fresh ginger

8- to 10-pound whole salmon, cleaned but
   with skin, head, and tail left on
Salt and freshly ground black pepper
Fresh herbs, for garnish

Pour the wine into a fish poacher or a covered pan fitted with a rack. Squeeze the juice from 1 lemon into the wine and add the fresh ginger. Slice the other lemon and place in the cavity of the fish along with salt and pepper. Place the fish on the rack, *not* in the liquid. Cover and bring the liquid to a boil, steaming the fish for 15 minutes.

Lower the heat so the liquid is barely at a simmer. Steam the salmon for about 1½ hours, checking periodically that there is enough liquid in the pan. If necessary, add more wine. The salmon is cooked when a meat thermometer registers 150° F. Remove the rack from the poacher and place the fish on a serving platter. Quickly remove the skin from the top of the fish.

Reduce the pan juices over high heat until about 1 cup of thickened sauce remains. Spoon the delicious ginger wine sauce over the fish and enjoy. Garnish the platter with additional lemon slices and fresh herbs.

Broiled Sea Bass with "Candied" Tomatoes and Seared Escarole

PROTEINS/FATS AND VEGGIES; LEVEL ONE

❖

SERVES 4

My daughter-in-law, Caroline, made this for me for Mother's Day this year. When no one was looking, I licked my plate. It's great with Sautéed Fennel (page 96).

4 Chilean sea bass fillets
Olive oil
Salt and freshly ground black pepper

2 large heads escarole, coarsely chopped
16 "Candied" Tomatoes (page 76)

Preheat the broiler. Brush the fish with a little olive oil and sprinkle with salt and pepper. Place the fish on a broiling pan and broil until golden brown and just cooked through the center, approximately 4 minutes per side. Cooking time will vary depending on the thickness of the fish.

Heat a large skillet or wok over high heat. Add a little olive oil and sauté the escarole until tender, about 4 minutes. Sprinkle with salt and pepper. Arrange on 4 plates. Place the sea bass on top of the escarole and top each piece of fish with 4 tomatoes.

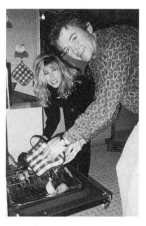

Cooking with Patrick Duffy, my favorite
Step by Step costar.

Fillet of Sole with Lemon-Caper Butter and Seared Spinach

PROTEINS/FATS AND VEGGIES; LEVEL ONE

SERVES 2

I cooked these in Brittany, France, with sole fresh from the North Atlantic Ocean—and I mean fresh! Alan and Jean Pierre went out in the boat after breakfast, and by lunchtime the fish were sizzling in the pan. Yum!

SOLE

1 tablespoon olive oil
2 large fillets of sole
¼ cup chicken broth (page 125)
1 tablespoon butter
2 tablespoons drained capers
2 tablespoons finely chopped parsley, plus
   additional for garnish
Juice from 1½ lemons

SEARED SPINACH

1 tablespoon olive oil
1 pound fresh spinach, torn, rinsed, and
   spun dry
Salt and freshly ground black pepper

For the sole: Heat a sauté pan large enough for both pieces of fish over high heat. Add the olive oil, then the fish, and sauté about 3 minutes per side. Remove the fish and set aside. With the heat still on high, add the chicken broth and reduce by half. Turn off the heat and stir in the butter until well combined. Stir in the capers, parsley, and half of the lemon juice. Set aside.

For the spinach: Heat a wok or large skillet over high heat. Add 1 teaspoon of the olive oil, then the spinach. Sauté for about a minute, until just wilted. Sprinkle with salt and pepper. Arrange on 2 plates.

Return the pan with the sauce to medium heat. Place the fish back in the pan to reheat, spooning the sauce over the fish. Serve the fish over the spinach with remaining lemon juice and olive oil on top. Garnish with fresh parsley.

Grilled Yellowfin Tuna with Tomato, Fennel, and Citrus Zest

PROTEINS/FATS AND VEGGIES; LEVEL ONE

SERVES 4

Fresh tuna is a little expensive, but it's worth it.

1 tablespoon olive oil
½ cup chopped onion
1 fennel bulb, sliced (reserve green tops
    for garnish)
2 garlic cloves, pressed
1 can (4½ ounces) plum tomatoes with
    juice

½ teaspoon fennel seeds
3 strips lemon zest
3 strips orange zest
Salt and freshly ground black pepper
4 yellowfin tuna (*ahi*) steaks
4 thin lemon slices, for garnish

Heat a skillet over high heat. Add the olive oil, then the onion and fennel. Sauté until the onion is translucent, about 3 minutes. Add the garlic and sauté an additional minute. Add the tomatoes with their juice, the fennel seeds, and the lemon and orange zests. Bring to a boil, then lower the heat and simmer for 15 minutes. Add salt and pepper to taste. Set sauce aside.

Prepare a grill. Season the tuna steaks with salt and pepper. Over medium heat (or in a pan with a bit of olive oil), grill the fish until barely cooked through—a few minutes on each side, depending on the thickness of the steaks. Arrange the steaks on a platter and surround with sauce. Garnish with the fennel tops and a lemon slice on each tuna steak.

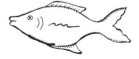

Roasted Trout with Lemon-Sage Mayonnaise

PROTEINS/FATS AND VEGGIES; LEVEL ONE

SERVES 4

Near our home in the desert is a trout farm. Corny as it may sound, it's really fun to go over there, throw a line in the water, and come home with dinner. This is delicious with steamed broccoli.

2 whole trout (1 pound each), butterflied
 and boned
Juice from 2 lemons
Salt and freshly ground black pepper
8 fresh sage leaves
2 to 3 tablespoons olive oil

GARNISH

8 lemon wedges
Fresh sage leaves
Lemon-Sage Mayonnaise (recipe follows)

Preheat the oven to 450°F.

Open each trout and season with some lemon juice, salt, pepper, and 4 sage leaves. Close the fish and rub olive oil and additional lemon juice on the exterior. Place in a roasting pan and bake for 15 to 20 minutes. Serve garnished with additional lemon wedges, fresh sage leaves, and a drizzle of Lemon-Sage Mayonnaise.

Lemon-Sage Mayonnaise

MAKES 1 CUP (ENOUGH FOR 4 SERVINGS OF FISH)

1 recipe Homemade Mayonnaise (page 86)
Juice from 1 lemon

1 teaspoon finely chopped fresh sage leaves
Freshly ground black pepper

Combine all the ingredients in a bowl. Cover and refrigerate to let the flavors mix.

Poultry

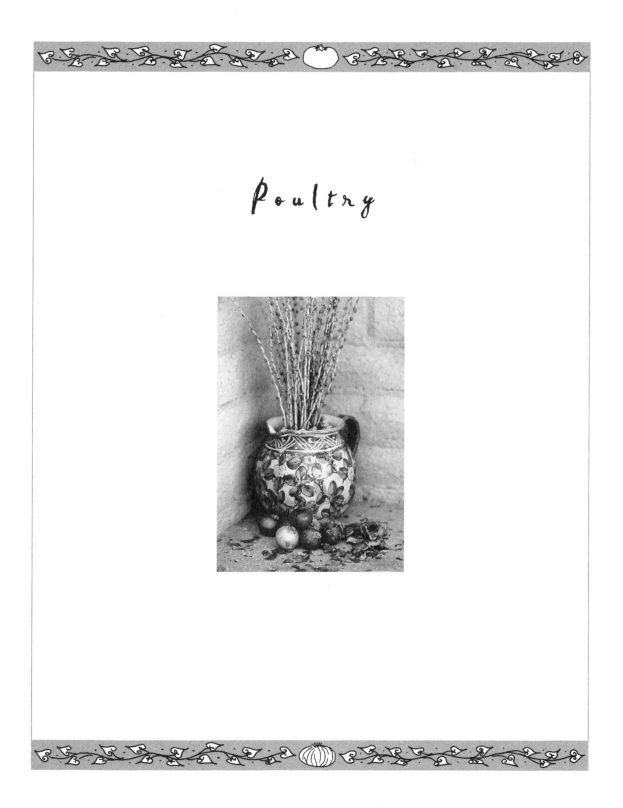

Chicken Piccata

SERVES 2

This is one of my favorite ways to eat chicken. It's light and lemony and yummy.

2 skinless and boneless chicken breasts
Salt and freshly ground black pepper
2 tablespoons olive oil
¼ cup white wine

2 tablespoons capers
Juice from 1 lemon
1 tablespoon butter

Rinse the chicken breasts and pat dry. Place each breast flat on a chopping block. With your knife parallel to the chopping block, slice the breast in half through the middle to make it half as thick. Place each slice between 2 layers of plastic wrap and pound with a mallet until ¼ inch thick. Season each breast with salt and pepper.

To a skillet over high heat, add the olive oil and as many of the chicken breasts as will fit in the pan without overlapping. Brown for 2 minutes on each side, then set aside in a warm oven.

To make the sauce, reheat the skillet over medium heat. Add the wine and reduce for 2 minutes or so, stirring constantly to scrape the brown bits off the bottom of the pan. Stir in the capers and the lemon juice. Remove from heat and add the butter, stirring until melted. Adjust salt and pepper to taste.

Pour the sauce over the chicken and serve. Great with steamed broccoli.

Roast Chicken with Mushroom Sausage Stuffing and Tarragon Gravy

PROTEINS/FATS AND VEGGIES; LEVEL ONE

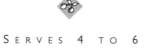

SERVES 4 TO 6

What a great Sunday night dinner! One of my children doesn't eat beef or pork, one doesn't eat fish, but they all like chicken. This is the family favorite.

1 recipe Mushroom Sausage Stuffing
   (page 167)
1 roasting chicken (5 to 6 pounds),
   washed well
2 tablespoons olive oil
2 bunches fresh tarragon
Salt and freshly ground black pepper
3 cups chicken broth

TARRAGON GRAVY

2 to 3 tablespoons pan drippings
2 cups dry white wine
2 tablespoons butter

Preheat the oven to 350° F. Place as much of the stuffing as will fit in the cavity of the chicken. Rub the outside of the chicken with olive oil, liberal amounts of tarragon, and salt and pepper. Pour the chicken broth in the bottom of a roasting pan. Add the chicken. Place a foil tent loosely over the chicken and bake for 1 hour. Remove the foil and cook for another 30 minutes.

Remove the cooked chicken and set aside. Pour off most of the fat in the pan, leaving 2 to 3 tablespoons to make the gravy.

For the gravy: Place the pan with the drippings on the stovetop over high heat.

Add the wine and stir, constantly scraping the bottom of the pan to incorporate the brown bits. When the liquid is reduced by half, lower the heat and add the butter, 1 tablespoon at a time, until well combined.

Remove the stuffing from the chicken and serve with the chicken and gravy.

Note An unstuffed chicken takes 20 minutes per pound to cook. Allow 25 minutes per pound for a stuffed chicken. You know the chicken is done when you prick the thigh with a fork and the juices run clear.

Lemon Roasted Chicken

SERVES 6

Healthy and low in fat, Lemon Roasted Chicken is a real crowd pleaser! These spicy, lemony skinless chicken legs were created by my son-in-law, Frank, who was born in Marseille, so the flavors are reminiscent of Southern France and Italy. Serve with bowls of steamed broccoli and cauliflower. Pour the lemony sauce over everything.

6 chicken legs, thighs attached
   (about 3 pounds)
2 medium yellow or sweet onions,
   quartered
6 lemons

10 garlic cloves, pressed
1 tablespoon dried rosemary or more
½ teaspoon cayenne pepper or more
Salt and freshly ground black pepper

Preheat the oven to 300° F.

Skin the chicken, if you like. Place the legs in a roasting pan with the quartered onions. Squeeze the juice from the lemons all over the chicken and then rub the pieces with garlic. Sprinkle on the rosemary, cayenne, salt, and pepper. Roast for about 90 minutes, or until cooked through.

To serve, pour the lemony garlic juices over the chicken and onions.

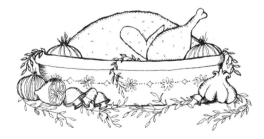

Clay Pot Chicken and Leeks

PROTEINS/FATS AND VEGGIES; LEVEL ONE

SERVES 4

I created this recipe while living in Las Vegas and starring nightly in the Moulin Rouge at the Hilton. Before I went to bed at four a.m., I would put the clay pot to soak in water. When I got up at noon, I would put all the ingredients in the clay pot, put it in the oven, and when I awoke from my afternoon nap, my house smelled like a gourmet chef was in the kitchen. This is sweet and juicy and delicious, and great served with Baked Garlic (page 80) to spread on the chicken.

4 large leeks, washed and halved, green tops removed
1 chicken (3 pounds), cut into pieces with skin removed
3 tablespoons ground cumin
Salt and freshly ground black pepper
3 tablespoons butter
3 cups chicken broth

If you have a clay pot, soak it in water overnight (or for at least 1 hour). If you don't have a clay pot, a Dutch oven will be fine.

Preheat the oven to 325°F. Line the bottom of the pot or Dutch oven with a layer of leeks. Then make a layer with pieces of chicken. Sprinkle the cumin, salt, and pepper over the chicken. Dot with a tablespoon of butter.

Begin layering again with leeks, chicken, cumin, salt, pepper, and butter. Over the top layer, put an additional layer of leeks. Pour in the broth and add any remaining butter. Cover and bake for 2 hours or until chicken is cooked through.

Chicken Paillard with Lemon-Parsley Butter and Seared Red Chard

PROTEINS/FATS AND VEGGIES; LEVEL ONE

SERVES 2

This takes less than 10 minutes to prepare—a simple, great meal to make after work. Fresh, delicious, and satisfying.

2 skinless and boneless chicken breasts
Salt and freshly ground black pepper
4 tablespoons olive oil
6 tablespoons unsalted butter
10 shallots, finely diced

Juice from 3 lemons
½ cup chicken broth
2 teaspoons chopped parsley
2 bunches red Swiss chard, coarsely
   chopped

Rinse the chicken breasts and pat dry. Place each breast flat on a chopping block. With your knife parallel to the chopping block, slice the breast in half through the middle to make it half as thick. Place each slice between 2 layers of plastic wrap and pound with a mallet until ¼ inch thick. Season each breast with salt and pepper.

Heat a skillet over high heat. Add 3 tablespoons of the olive oil and as many of the chicken slices as will fit in the pan without overlapping. Brown for 2 minutes on each side, then set aside on a shallow baking pan in an oven on warm. Repeat with remaining chicken.

Place the chicken pan over medium heat and melt 3 tablespoons of the butter. Add the shallots, cooking until soft, about 5 minutes. Add the lemon juice and chicken broth and bring to a boil. Reduce by half. Cut the remaining 3 tablespoons butter into small pieces and whisk into the pan until sauce is smooth. Remove from the heat. Stir in additional salt, pepper, and the parsley. Keep warm.

Heat a wok or large skillet over very high heat. Add the remaining tablespoon olive oil and the chard, quickly cooking until just wilted, about 1 minute. Season with salt and pepper. Arrange the chicken over the chard on a platter and top with the lemon butter sauce.

Chicken Paillard with Fresh Tomato Salsa and Arugula

PROTEINS/FATS AND VEGGIES; LEVEL ONE

❖

SERVES 4

These chicken breasts are sliced in half and pounded until they are nice and thin. The simple accompaniment of salsa and fresh arugula makes this dish light and satisfying on a hot summer night.

SALSA

4 medium tomatoes, diced
1 bunch flat-leaf parsley, chopped
2 garlic cloves, minced
2 tablespoons extra-virgin olive oil
Juice from ½ lemon
Salt and freshly ground black pepper

CHICKEN PAILLARD

4 skinless and boneless chicken breasts
Salt and freshly ground black pepper
2 sprigs fresh rosemary, chopped
    (or 2 tablespoons dried)
2 tablespoons olive oil

GARNISH

1 bunch fresh arugula (or your favorite green)

For the salsa: Combine the ingredients in a medium bowl and set aside to let the flavors combine. (Do not refrigerate or the tomatoes will get mealy.)

For the chicken: Rinse the chicken breasts and pat them dry. Place each breast flat on a chopping block and slice in half through the middle to make it half as thick (with your knife parallel to the chopping block). Place each slice between 2 layers of plastic wrap and pound with a mallet until the chicken is ¼ inch thick.

Season each breast with salt, pepper, and rosemary.

Heat a skillet over high heat. Add the olive oil and as many of the chicken pieces as will fit in the pan without overlapping. Brown for 2 to 3 minutes on each side and set aside in an oven on warm. Repeat for remaining chicken.

Line 4 dinner plates with fresh arugula. Arrange 2 pieces of chicken on top of the arugula on each plate and garnish each plate with a large spoonful of salsa.

Moroccan Chicken with Preserved Lemon Rinds

PROTEINS/FATS AND VEGGIES; LEVEL ONE

SERVES 8

This chicken is especially tender, with an exotic flavor. On Level Two you can make it with red Moroccan olives for truly authentic preparation. I usually find red olives at ethnic grocery stores or in the gourmet section of the market.

¼ cup olive oil
2 fryer chickens (3 pounds each), skinned
   and cut into serving pieces
4 cups water
4 garlic cloves, minced
3 medium onions, coarsely chopped
1 cup chopped fresh cilantro

1 cup chopped fresh parsley
4 teaspoons ground cumin
1 teaspoon ground ginger
½ teaspoon saffron
½ teaspoon salt
2 Preserved Lemon Rinds, thinly sliced
   (opposite)

Heat the olive oil in a Dutch oven or a large pot with a lid. Add the chicken pieces and brown on both sides over high heat. Pour in the water. Add the garlic, onions, cilantro, parsley, cumin, ginger, saffron, and salt. Lower the heat, cover, and simmer for 1 hour.

Remove the chicken pieces, reserving them on a platter. Turn the heat back up to high until the liquid boils and reduce by one third. Add the preserved lemon rinds and reduce the heat. Place the chicken pieces back in the sauce to reheat.

For Level Two
Add 1 cup of red olives at the same time you add the preserved lemons. You can substitute Greek olives if red are unavailable, but the red olives are especially tasty.

Preserved Lemon Rinds

Preserved lemons—a Level One food—are something I make on a regular basis. This simple process removes any bitterness from the lemon rind and creates a uniquely sweet yet tart flavor. I love the way they look, beautifully displayed in glass jars on the kitchen counter.

Lemons
Kosher salt, 1 to 2 tablespoons per lemon
Water

Thoroughly wash as many lemons as you care to make. Set each lemon on a cutting board with the stem side up. Slice in half, lengthwise, down to the bottom without cutting all the way through. Then slice again, almost down to the bottom, creating a quartered lemon that opens like a flower.

Pour the salt liberally inside each lemon.

Gently close each lemon and put them in a clean jar with a lid that seals tightly. Fill the jar with as many lemons as will easily fit. Add water to the top of the jar, seal, and let sit for 30 days.

Remove the lemons one at a time. Scoop out the insides and discard. Slice the remaining lemon rind into desired sizes.

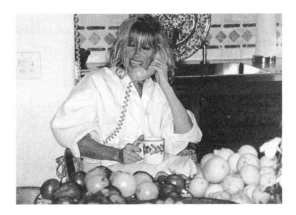

Alan bought too much produce again!

Roasted Herbes de Provence Chicken

PROTEINS/FATS AND VEGGIES; LEVEL ONE

SERVES 4 TO 6

This can be made for Sunday night dinner with the family and the leftovers eaten in different forms the rest of the week. Use the leftover chicken meat for Tarragon Chicken Salad in Lettuce Cups (page 118). And then make my yummy Chicken Tomato Cilantro Soup (page 126) with the carcass. Remember to save all drippings and juices to use for sauces, soups, or stews.

1 chicken (5 to 6 pounds)
2 to 3 tablespoons olive oil
Salt and freshly ground black pepper
3 tablespoons herbes de Provence
1 large bunch fresh tarragon

3 yellow onions, roughly chopped
2 parsnips, peeled and roughly chopped
1 cup chicken broth
1 cup dry white wine
1 tablespoon butter

Preheat the oven to 350°F.

Remove the giblets from the chicken. Rinse the bird and pat it dry. Place it in a roasting pan and rub with some of the olive oil. Season with salt, pepper, and herbes de Provence. Place the tarragon under the skin, in the cavity, and all around the outside of the bird. Place one of the chopped onions in the cavity. Sprinkle the remaining onions and parsnips around the chicken in the pan. Drizzle a little more oil on the vegetables. Pour the broth in the bottom of the pan. Put a foil tent on top of the chicken, and bake for 1 hour. Remove the tent and let brown for another 30 to 40 minutes. The total cooking time is about 20 minutes per pound.

Remove the chicken from the roasting pan and place it on a serving platter. Pour off most of the fat from the pan, reserving 2 to 3 tablespoons. Place the roasting pan on the stove and heat the drippings over high heat. Add the wine and scrape the brown bits off the bottom of the pan to make a sauce. Reduce for 5 to 7 minutes, or until desired thickness is achieved. Adjust seasonings to taste with salt and pepper. Turn off the heat and add the butter. Stir until well combined. Carve the chicken and serve with a spoonful of sauce.

Chicken with Forty Cloves of Garlic

PROTEINS/FATS AND VEGGIES; LEVEL ONE

SERVES 4

Eat this dinner with good friends! After your delicious meal, pour the carcass, juices, and leftovers in a soup pot, cover with water, bring to a boil, then simmer for 6 hours in a stockpot. Now you have soup for tomorrow's dinner.

1 chicken (5 pounds)
6 tablespoons olive oil
Salt and freshly ground black pepper
3 sprigs fresh thyme
2 sprigs fresh rosemary
3 sprigs fresh sage

40 garlic cloves, unpeeled
3 sprigs flat-leaf parsley
10 whole black peppercorns
1 cup chicken broth, or more as needed
1 cup dry white wine

Preheat the oven to 400°F.

Rub the outside of the chicken with olive oil. Season inside and out with salt and pepper. Put half the thyme, rosemary, and sage, plus 5 garlic cloves in the cavity of the chicken. Place the chicken in a Dutch oven fitted with a lid (or use a roasting pan and later cover tightly with foil). Scatter the remaining thyme, rosemary, sage, and garlic, and the parsley and peppercorns around the bird. Pour the broth in the bottom of the pan. Cover and bake for approximately 1 hour, then remove the cover or foil and let the bird brown for another 30 to 40 minutes. The total cooking time is about 20 minutes per pound of chicken.

Remove the chicken from the pan and place it on a serving platter with the garlic spread all around. Put the pan with the drippings on the stovetop over high heat. Add the wine and scrape up any browned bits from the bottom of the pan, stirring constantly to reduce the sauce until it starts to thicken. If most of the drippings have evaporated, add another ½ cup of broth and reduce. Adjust salt and pepper to taste.

Carve the meat and serve with a spoonful of sauce and a few cloves of garlic. The garlic will easily slip out of the skins and add a delicious flavor to the chicken.

Thanksgiving Turkey with Mushroom Sausage Stuffing and Tarragon Gravy

PROTEINS/FATS AND VEGGIES; LEVEL ONE

SERVES 12 TO 14

Once you've made this recipe for turkey, stuffing, and gravy, you'll never go back to the traditional again.

1 turkey (14 pounds)
Mushroom Sausage Stuffing (opposite)
6 tablespoons butter, softened

2 bunches fresh tarragon, chopped
Salt and freshly ground black pepper
8 cups chicken broth

Preheat the oven to 325°F.

Fill the cavity of the turkey with stuffing. Rub the outside of the turkey with 3 tablespoons of the butter, the tarragon, salt, and pepper. Pour 6 cups of broth into the bottom of the roasting pan.

Bake the turkey for about 4 hours, basting every 30 minutes or so. If the bird starts getting too brown, cover with a foil tent. (Check for doneness with a meat thermometer—it should register somewhere between 162°F and 170°F.) When the turkey is cooked, remove it from the pan and keep warm.

Pour off most of the fat in the roasting pan, until only 2 to 3 tablespoons remain. Heat the remaining 2 cups of broth. Place the roasting pan on the stovetop over high heat and add the hot broth, scraping the brown bits off the bottom of the pan. Reduce by half and remove from the heat. Add the remaining butter, one tablespoon at a time, until well combined. Carve the turkey and serve with the stuffing and delicious tarragon-flavored gravy. Be sure to put lots of sauce on the plate so the other side dishes are flavored by these great-tasting juices.

Mushroom Sausage Stuffing

This is the most incredible stuffing for your Thanksgiving turkey or roast chicken. You can use it in stuffed Provençal vegetables (see pages 102–104) or just have it as a side dish. No one will ever ask for bread stuffing again.

4 onions, thinly sliced
2 to 4 tablespoons olive oil
4 cups coarsely chopped shiitake and oyster
   mushrooms (or regular white button
   mushrooms)
Salt and freshly ground black pepper

½ cup dry white wine
2 tablespoons butter
2 pounds spicy turkey sausage meat,
   removed from casings
1 bunch fresh tarragon, leaves only

Sauté the onions in olive oil over medium-low heat until caramelized, about 30 minutes. Turn the heat up to medium-high and add the mushrooms. Sauté the mushrooms until crisp on the edges, about 10 to 15 minutes. Season with salt and pepper. Turn the heat to high and add the wine. Let the wine cook off for a couple of minutes, then lower the heat and simmer with the mushrooms for another 10 minutes. Stir in the butter 1 tablespoon at a time until combined. Remove from the heat and set aside.

In large skillet, brown the sausage. When cooked through, about 5 to 7 minutes, add to the mushroom mixture along with the tarragon and combine thoroughly.

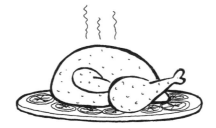

Turkey Meatloaf

SERVES 4

Great with Celery Root Puree (page 98) and steamed string beans!

1 pound ground turkey
   (or beef, if you prefer)
1 egg yolk
3 tablespoons chopped parsley
1 tablespoon butter, softened
½ medium onion, chopped

1 teaspoon lemon juice
1 teaspoon salt
1 teaspoon freshly ground black pepper
1 cup chicken broth
   (or beef broth if using ground beef)

Preheat the oven to 350°F.

In a large mixing bowl, combine all ingredients except the broth. Form into a loaf and place in a lightly greased loaf pan.

Pour the broth over the top and bake for 1 hour, basting periodically. When finished, cut into slices and spoon the juices from the bottom of the pan over the meat.

Turkey Sausage with Peppers and Onions

PROTEINS/FATS AND VEGGIES; LEVEL ONE

SERVES 6

This recipe is so easy, and it's packed with flavor.

2 large yellow or sweet onions, thinly sliced
4 green or red bell peppers, julienned

¼ cup olive oil
12 hot turkey sausages (or your favorite)

In a large sauté pan over medium heat, cook the onions and peppers in olive oil, stirring frequently until the peppers are soft and the onions are caramelized, about 30 minutes. Cook the sausages on a grill or brown them in a skillet and serve them atop a heaping mound of peppers and onions.

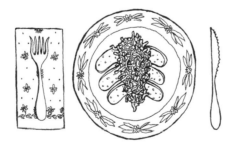

Turkey Cutlet with Classic Marinara Sauce

PROTEINS/FATS AND VEGGIES; LEVEL ONE

SERVES 4

These are wonderful served with Seared Spinach (page 152).

MARINARA SAUCE

2 tablespoons olive oil
1 medium onion, chopped
4 garlic cloves, pressed
1 can (28 ounces) tomato sauce
2 tablespoons chopped parsley
1 teaspoon dried basil
½ teaspoon dried oregano

TURKEY CUTLET

4 turkey cutlets (slices of turkey breast)
1 tablespoon dried rosemary
1 teaspoon dried thyme
Salt and freshly ground black pepper
4 tablespoons olive oil

For the marinara sauce: Heat the olive oil in a saucepan. Add the onion and cook until translucent, approximately 5 minutes. Add the garlic and cook 1 minute longer. Add the tomato sauce and herbs and bring to a boil. Lower the heat and simmer for 1 hour or more.

For the turkey: Season the cutlets with the rosemary, thyme, salt, and pepper. Heat the olive oil in a large skillet over medium-high heat. Add the turkey cutlets—as many as will fit without overlapping. Brown the cutlets on both sides and continue cooking until cooked through, approximately 4 minutes per side, depending on thickness of cutlet. Cover and keep warm. Repeat with remaining cutlets.

Serve the cutlets topped with marinara sauce.

Confit of Duck

SERVES 4 TO 6

Got all day? In the mood to cook? Well, this recipe is very time-consuming but once completed provides the best "fast food" ever. The duck will keep in the refrigerator for up to eight weeks and needs only a quick reheat for an amazing meal any time. Don't be startled by the amount of fat used in the cooking process. All the fat in the duck cooks off in this age-old technique of slow-cooking duck in its rendered fat. You're left with the most tender, greaseless duck you've ever eaten.

2 ducks (5 pounds each), quartered (4 legs with thighs attached, 4 breasts); reserve remaining wings, neck, and bones for stock
1 cup kosher salt
2 tablespoons cracked black peppercorns
¼ cup mixed dried herbs (thyme, marjoram, bay leaf)
½ tablespoon allspice berries, crushed
½ tablespoon juniper berries, crushed
8 cups solid (unrendered) duck fat
6 garlic cloves

Rinse the ducks and pat dry. Combine the salt, pepper, herbs, and spices in a bowl. Coat each piece of duck in the mixture and lay flat in a dish, sprinkling the remainder of the salt mixture on top. Refrigerate for at least 2 hours (even better, up to 24 hours).

To render the fat, put the solid fat and the fatty duck skin in a pot with five times the amount of water as duck fat. Bring to a boil and simmer for 2 hours. Do not let the water boil away. Strain and refrigerate the fat and water until the fat is hard. Lift off the fat and discard the water. If you are short on duck fat, you can supplement with chicken fat, pork fat, or even olive oil.

Wipe the duck pieces free of salt. Melt the rendered fat in a Dutch oven and put the duck pieces in it close together so that the duck is covered with the fat. Add the garlic and simmer very gently until the duck is tender, 1½ to 2 hours. When pierced with a fork, the duck should fall off the fork when shaken.

Transfer the duck to a baking dish and add the fat. (Try not to bring any juice with the duck.) The duck should be completely covered with the fat. It will stay preserved in the fat for up to 8 weeks in the refrigerator. To serve, lift the duck out of the fat, then remove and discard any skin or extra fat. Reheat in a 400° F. oven for 15 minutes and serve immediately.

Meat

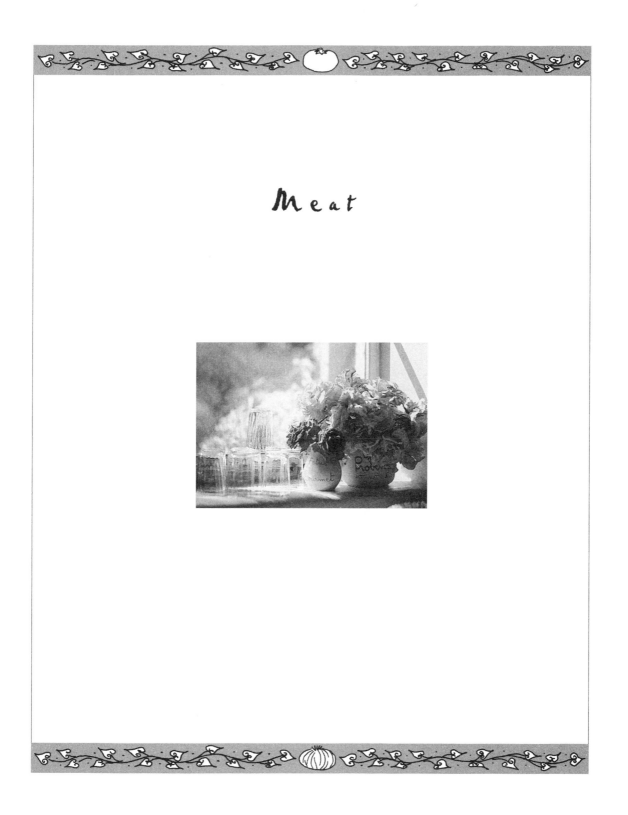

Grilled Pepper Steak with Herb Butter

PROTEINS/FATS AND VEGGIES; LEVEL ONE

SERVES 2 TO 3

This is a great recipe to make on the grill. Serve it with Vegetables Provençal (page 92) and Celery Root Puree (page 98). Piercing the steak with a fork before brushing it with olive oil makes the meat tender and gives it great flavor.

1 New York strip steak (2 pounds),
   trimmed of fat
3 tablespoons olive oil
4 tablespoons black peppercorns
4 garlic cloves, minced

Salt to taste
2 tablespoons butter
1 teaspoon finely chopped fresh basil
1 teaspoon finely chopped fresh thyme

Heat grill to high. Pierce the steaks all over with a fork—at least 8 times—to let the oil penetrate. Rub with olive oil.

Crack the peppercorns with the bottom of a heavy saucepan. Combine with the garlic and salt to make a paste. Cover both sides of the steaks with the mixture.

For medium rare to medium steaks, cook on a hot grill for 4 to 5 minutes per side. Remove from heat and set aside for 10 minutes.

Melt the butter in a saucepan and add the herbs. Slice the steaks on the diagonal and drizzle with herb butter.

Beef Stir-Fry with Fragrant Vegetables

PROTEINS/FATS AND VEGGIES; LEVEL ONE

SERVES 4

When Alan was growing up, his mother ran a boarding house, where she took care of a family of seven Chinese brothers. Alan's "Chinese brother" Dick gave us this recipe. By the way, Alan was nine years old before he realized Santa was not necessarily Chinese.

¾ pound boneless sirloin, trimmed of fat
    and cut into ¼-inch strips
2 tablespoons finely chopped fresh ginger
2 garlic cloves, minced
½ cup beef broth
2 tablespoons soy sauce

2 tablespoons vegetable oil
2 cups broccoli florets
1 yellow squash, sliced
1 red bell pepper, julienned
4 green onions, sliced on the diagonal
¼ teaspoon hot red pepper flakes

Marinate the beef strips for at least 1 hour in a mixture of the ginger, garlic, broth, soy sauce, and vegetable oil.

Heat a wok or large skillet over high heat. Add 1 tablespoon vegetable oil and the broccoli. Cook the broccoli for about 5 minutes. Add the squash and stir-fry for an additional 2 to 3 minutes. Add the bell pepper and cook 1 to 2 more minutes. Remove the vegetables and set aside.

Add another tablespoon of vegetable oil, the beef strips, including the marinade, and cook over high heat for a minute or two, until just cooked through. Stir the vegetables back into the wok to reheat, adding the green onions and red pepper flakes. After about 1 minute, remove from the heat. Serve immediately.

For Level Two
Serve over brown rice.

Greek Beef Kabobs

MAKES ABOUT 8 KABOBS

These kabobs are great for summer grilling. This recipe calls for beef, but any of your favorite meats will work well. You can find metal or wooden skewers in your local grocery store. This is excellent with Greek Salad (page 113).

1 pound boneless sirloin steak, cut into
   2-inch cubes
¼ cup olive oil
1 tablespoon dried oregano
Salt and freshly ground black pepper

24 pearl onions, peeled
24 cherry tomatoes, stems removed
3 red or green bell peppers, seeded and
   chopped into 2-inch squares
24 mushrooms, stems removed

Place the sirloin, olive oil, oregano, salt, and pepper in a noncorrosive bowl. Marinate in the refrigerator at least 1 hour or as long as overnight. Drain and reserve the marinade for basting.

Prepare a grill. To make the kabobs, skewer the meat and vegetables in a pretty pattern. Repeat the process until your skewer is full. Thread the next kabob and continue until all your ingredients are used up.

Over very high heat, lay the kabobs on the grill and cook, basting with leftover marinade, until the meat is done to your liking, 6 minutes for medium.

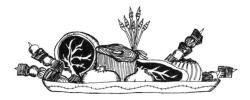

Grilled Lamb Chops with Fresh Herbs

PROTEINS/FATS AND VEGGIES; LEVEL ONE

SERVES 6

On Alan's birthday every year, he asks me to make these lamb chops, scrambled eggs, and fresh asparagus. Sweet and tasty, they make a great breakfast, lunch, or dinner.

½ cup olive oil
6 garlic cloves, chopped
½ cup red wine
1 bunch fresh rosemary, chopped
2 tablespoons chopped fresh thyme

18 baby lamb chops, 1 inch thick
Salt and freshly ground black pepper
Fresh rosemary and thyme sprigs, for
    garnish

In a noncorrosive dish, mix the oil, garlic, wine, and herbs. Add the lamb chops and marinate 4 hours, turning the chops after 2 hours to marinate both sides.

Prepare a grill. Season the lamb chops with salt and pepper. Grill over high heat until medium rare, 2 to 3 minutes per side. Arrange on a platter in a fan pattern and garnish with rosemary and thyme sprigs.

Medallions of Lamb

PROTEINS/FATS AND VEGGIES; LEVEL ONE

SERVES 6

This takes only 20 minutes to make and is unbelievably good. It's a great recipe to prepare for company. Make the sauce ahead of time, and all you have to do when you are ready to eat is sauté the lamb for 2 minutes on each side and serve.

2 racks of lamb, boned and trimmed
4 tablespoons ground cumin
2 tablespoons butter
4 tablespoons olive oil
12 to 15 shallots, chopped

6 garlic cloves, chopped
6 ripe medium tomatoes, chopped
Salt and freshly ground black pepper
1 bunch fresh basil leaves, julienned

Slice the fillet of lamb into ½-inch medallions. Rub both sides of the medallions generously with cumin. Set aside.

Heat a large sauté pan over medium heat. Add the butter, 2 tablespoons of the olive oil, and the shallots. Sauté the shallots until they are lightly browned, about 2 minutes. Add the garlic and cook for 1 minute longer. Add the tomatoes, salt, and pepper. Lower the heat and simmer for 5 minutes.

In another pan, sauté the lamb medallions in the remaining 2 tablespoons olive oil for approximately 2 minutes on each side. Just before serving, toss the basil into the tomato sauce and pour over the lamb medallions. Serve immediately.

Curried Lamb with Cucumber-Mint Sour Cream in Radicchio Cups

PROTEINS/FATS AND VEGGIES; LEVEL ONE

❖

SERVES 8

This is a great lunch, or served hot or cold as appetizers at a cocktail party. Everyone loves this recipe —except my vegetarian friends.

CURRIED LAMB

2 tablespoons olive oil
1 medium onion, chopped
2 garlic cloves, chopped
1 pound ground lamb (from leg)
1 tablespoon curry powder
½ teaspoon ground cinnamon
Salt and freshly ground pepper

CUCUMBER-MINT SOUR CREAM

½ medium cucumber, peeled, seeded, and diced
¼ cup chopped fresh mint
⅓ cup sour cream
Juice from 2 limes

RADICCHIO CUPS

8 radicchio leaves
8 mint leaves, for garnish

For the lamb: Heat a large sauté pan over medium heat. Add the olive oil and onion, and cook until the onion is golden brown, about 5 minutes. Add the garlic and cook for 1 minute more. Add the lamb, and season the meat with the curry powder, cinnamon, salt, and pepper. Sauté over medium-high heat until the lamb is cooked through, about 15 minutes, and set aside.

For the sour cream: Place all the ingredients into a bowl and mix them until well combined.

Fill each radicchio leaf with a large spoonful of curried lamb. Top with sour cream sauce and garnish with a mint leaf. Fold up like a taco and enjoy.

Minted Lamb in Cucumber Boats with Marinated Red Onions

PROTEINS/FATS AND VEGGIES; LEVEL ONE

MAKES 12 SMALL BOATS; SERVES 4 AS A LIGHT LUNCH
OR 6 AS APPETIZERS

This spicy lamb is served in cool cucumber boats with tangy and sweet marinated red onions. It makes a wonderful hot or cold lunch or cocktail appetizer. It includes many wonderful traditional Thai flavors, including a sauce which can be found in Asian markets.

MARINATED RED ONIONS

1 medium red onion, sliced paper thin
Juice from 6 limes
Salt

6 small pickling cucumbers, such as Kirby

MINTED LAMB

2 tablespoons olive oil
3 serrano chilies, seeded and finely
   chopped
1 tablespoon minced ginger
4 garlic cloves, chopped
¾ pound ground lamb (from leg)
1 tablespoon Thai fish sauce (optional)
Freshly ground black pepper
3 tablespoons chopped fresh mint
Juice from 2 limes

For the red onions: Place the red onion in a bowl with the juice from 6 limes and a pinch of salt. Let stand for a few hours.

Cut the cucumbers in half lengthwise. Scoop out a good portion of the center with a spoon or a melon baller, creating a boat shape to hold the lamb filling. (I like the skin of unwaxed cucumbers, so I leave it on. If you don't like it, peel the skin off before you cut the cucumber.) Set aside in refrigerator.

For the lamb filling: Heat a sauté pan over medium heat. Add the oil, then the chilies. Cook for 2 to 3 minutes. Add the ginger and garlic and cook until golden brown. Add the lamb and brown over medium-high heat, seasoning with the fish sauce and pepper. When the meat is cooked through, about 10 minutes, remove from the heat and toss with the mint and juice from 2 limes.

Fill the cucumber boats with the minted lamb and top with marinated onions.

Pork Medallions with Pepper-Thyme Vinaigrette

PROTEINS/FATS AND VEGGIES; LEVEL ONE

❖

SERVES 4

Pork is one of those ignored meats. What I like about it is that it's a flavor carrier—the taste of the meat is so mild that it picks up whatever flavoring you add to it. This makes a great summer meal— cool lettuce, warm pork, with a tangy peppery dressing.

PORK MEDALLIONS

2 pork tenderloins
½ cup olive oil
Juice from 1 lemon
2 teaspoons fresh thyme

1 head Bibb lettuce, leaves separated,
    washed, and dried
2 heads frisée (baby curly endive), washed
    and dried
1½ cups cherry tomatoes

PEPPER-THYME VINAIGRETTE

Juice from 2 lemons
1 teaspoon salt
½ cup extra-virgin olive oil
¼ cup black peppercorns
6 shallots, very finely chopped
1 teaspoon fresh thyme

For the pork: Rinse and pat dry the tenderloins. Slice on the diagonal into ¼-inch medallions. Place them in a noncorrosive container and marinate in the olive oil, lemon juice, and thyme. Cover and refrigerate for 2 hours, turning after 1 hour.

For the vinaigrette: Place the lemon juice in a small bowl. Add the salt, then the olive oil in a thin, steady stream, whisking constantly. Set aside about a third of the lemon oil. On a chopping block, crack the peppercorns using a frying pan. Add the cracked peppercorns, shallots, and thyme to the remaining lemon oil.

In a hot frying pan over medium-high heat, cook the marinated pork approximately 2 minutes per side (do not overcook, or it will get dry and tough). The pork should be just cooked through, juicy with a hint of pink in the center.

Toss the lettuce with the reserved lemon oil. Arrange on 4 plates. Fan the pork medallions on the lettuce and top with a generous amount of the vinaigrette. Garnish with cherry tomatoes and serve immediately.

Traditional Mexican Carnitas

PROTEINS/FATS AND VEGGIES; LEVEL ONE

SERVES 6

Because I live in Southern California, my cooking has been greatly influenced by Mexican cuisine. This recipe is normally served with corn tortillas, but I like to pile the crispy cooked pork into iceberg lettuce cups with lots of salsa.

1 piece pork shoulder (3 pounds),
   skinned and boned
2 teaspoons salt
1 head iceberg lettuce

Spicy Tomato Salsa (page 143,
   or a prepared version)
1 container (16 ounces) sour cream

Cut the pork with the fat into strips about 2¾ inches thick. Place the strips in a large, shallow skillet and sprinkle with the salt. Barely cover with cold water and bring to a boil, uncovered. Lower the heat to medium and let the meat continue cooking briskly until all the liquid has evaporated— by this time it should be cooked through, but not falling apart. Turn the heat down to medium low and continue cooking until all the fat has rendered out of the pork. The pork will begin to brown in its own juices. Keep turning until it is browned all over, about 70 minutes. The pork is done when it is a little crispy and shredding into pieces.

Remove the iceberg leaves from the head in whole pieces. Rinse and dry. Place a spoonful of meat in each lettuce leaf. Serve with salsa and sour cream. Fold up like a taco and enjoy.

For Level Two

If you want to wrap the carnitas in a tortilla, use a whole wheat tortilla instead of a white flour or corn tortilla. Or try them with my Black Bean Chili (page 143). Either way, you're mixing Proteins/Fats with Carbos, so make sure you correct this imbalance by eating Level One meals until you get your balance back.

Osso Buco

SERVES 6

This is a good meal to make on a Sunday. You can nibble on it all week long.

2 tablespoons olive oil
1 meaty veal shank, split into 6 pieces
  (approximately 3 pounds)
2 cups chicken broth
½ cup diced zucchini
½ cup diced red onion
½ cup diced celery
½ cup diced parsnips
2 garlic cloves, finely chopped
Salt and freshly ground black pepper
3 tablespoons tomato paste
¼ cup finely chopped flat-leaf parsley

Heat a Dutch oven over medium-high heat. Add the olive oil and veal. Brown veal for about 5 minutes on each side, then stack on one side of the pot. Add 1 cup of the broth. Bring to a boil and add the zucchini, onion, celery, parsnips, and garlic. Lower the heat and cook until the liquid reduces, about 5 minutes. Arrange the veal pieces over the vegetables and sprinkle with salt and pepper.

In a small saucepan, heat the remaining cup of broth. Stir in the tomato paste and add to the veal. Cover and simmer for 40 minutes. Remove the veal and puree the vegetables and broth with a hand mixer (or transfer to a food processor). Serve the veal in shallow bowls surrounded with the pureed sauce. Garnish with parsley.

Desserts

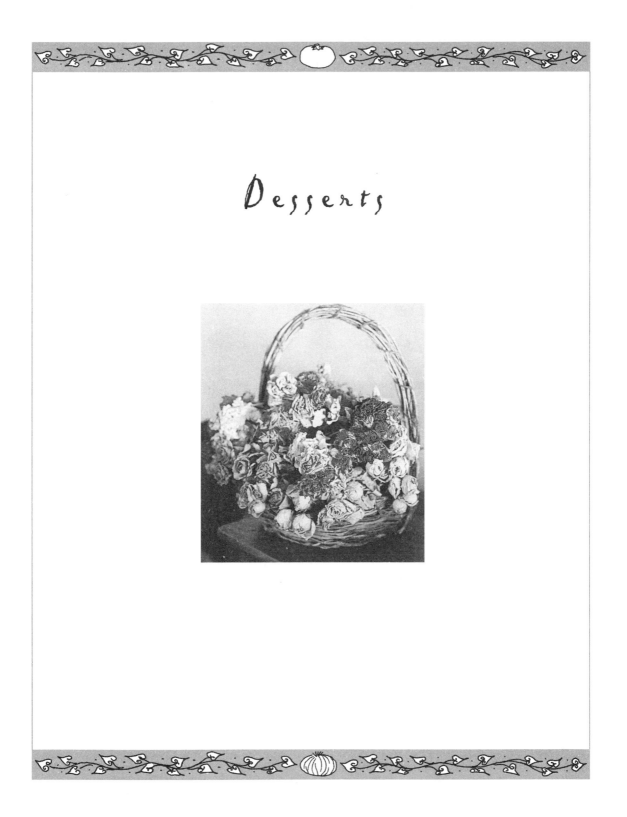

Sugarless Cheesecake

PROTEINS/FATS; LEVEL ONE

SERVES 6

I created this recipe for my Auntie Helen, who is diabetic and cannot have any sugar. I was surprised at how great it tasted with no sugar and no flour. But although it may be fine for diabetics, I don't recommend it for heart patients or those on cholesterol-restricted diets!

2 packages (8 ounces each) cream cheese
12 packets NutraSweet
3 large eggs
3 tablespoons fresh lemon juice

1½ teaspoons vanilla extract
¼ teaspoon salt
3 cups sour cream
Mint sprigs or rose petals, for garnish

Preheat the oven to 350°F.

In a large mixing bowl, beat the cream cheese and sweetener until very smooth, about 3 minutes. Add the eggs, one at a time, beating well after each addition. Add the lemon juice, vanilla, and salt. Beat in the sour cream until just blended.

Grease an 8-inch springform pan with 2½-inch sides and line the bottom with greased parchment or waxed paper. Wrap the outside of the pan with a double layer of heavy-duty foil to prevent seepage.

Pour the batter into the pan. Set the pan in a large roasting pan and surround with 1 inch of very hot water. Bake for 45 minutes. Turn off the oven without opening the door and let the cake cool 1 hour.

Remove to a rack and cool to room temperature, about 1 hour. Cover with plastic wrap and refrigerate overnight. Unmold the cake onto a plate and garnish with mint.

For Level Two
Spoon the following delicious sauce around the cheesecake.

Raspberry Sauce

1 package frozen raspberries, thawed
3 to 4 packets NutraSweet

1 teaspoon lemon juice

Combine all ingredients in a blender or food processor until pureed.

Decaf Coffee Granita

LEVEL ONE

SERVES 6

Granita is like a shaved ice—cool and refreshing. This recipe may be eaten after any meal in Level One because it is made with only decaf coffee and artificial sweetener. If you're having a Proteins/Fats meal, for a great treat you can top this dessert with some whipped cream.

8 cups strong decaf coffee (for best results, use decaf espresso), cooled
6 packets NutraSweet, or to taste

OPTIONAL GARNISH

1 pint heavy cream
1 teaspoon vanilla extract

Combine the cooled coffee and the NutraSweet in a metal bowl. Place the bowl in the freezer. Every 30 minutes, open the freezer and use a metal whisk to stir the coffee, removing any frozen pieces from the side of the bowl. You will probably see the first frozen pieces after a couple of hours. Be sure to keep whisking your granita every 30 minutes until you are ready to serve it, or it will become one large ice block. After about 3 hours, the granita will be nicely frozen and ready to serve.

To make the whipped cream, place the cream and vanilla in a bowl. (Add NutraSweet if you like your whipped cream sweet.) Beat with a whisk or an electric mixer until soft peaks form. Spoon granita into cups or glasses and top with whipped cream.

CHAPTER TWELVE

Level Two: Keep on Cookin'!

Level Two is all about maintaining your weight, which means straying from Level One guidelines only as much as your body can handle. Enjoy any of the Level One dishes from the previous section but try preparing them in the Level Two variations.

Additionally, in this section, I have included a few special recipes that are specific to Level Two. Many of them are Carbo and Veggies recipes in which there is some added fat. These include delicious meals like Whole Wheat Pasta with Pine Nuts, White Bean Garden Salad, and my stunning-looking and -tasting "Candied" Tomato Tart. (But you still won't find a potato in the batch.)

I've also included a number of Level Two desserts. These are perfectly suitable for company and taste lavish without creating as much of an imbalance in your system as their conventional counterparts. For ex-

ample, my Decadent Chocolate Cake is fudgy and rich, made with dark chocolate, eggs, butter, cream, and a touch of whole wheat flour and sugar. It's not health food, but it's much better for Somersizing purposes than a boxed cake mix, loaded with sugar, white flour, and chemicals. The desserts in this book are made with whole wheat flour and a reduced amount of sugar without affecting flavor.

This isn't to say, however, that you should sit down and polish off a whole Decadent Chocolate Cake. The key to maintaining your weight is moderation. When I want to have dessert, I usually eat a Level One meal and then enjoy a luscious treat.

Have fun in Level Two. Soon you'll be creating your own recipes and sharing them with your friends. I hope you'll send me a copy, too!

"Candied" Tomato Tart

LEVEL TWO

MAKES 6 APPETIZERS OR ABOUT 3 ENTRÉES
WITH A GREEN SALAD

This tart is made with phyllo dough, which can be found in the freezer section of many grocery stores. Most phyllo doughs are made with whole wheat, which makes this delicious tart a lovely option on Level Two. I made this for dinner along with a salad, and Alan and I almost finished the entire thing!

5 to 6 sheets phyllo dough
¼ cup olive oil
24 "Candied" Tomato halves (page 76)

Preheat the oven to 350° F. Thaw the phyllo dough.

Put one layer of phyllo on a cookie sheet and brush lightly with olive oil. Fold in the ends to create an edge for your tart, securing with a little more olive oil. (I make a 9 × 6-inch tart, but you can make any shape or size you like by cutting the phyllo dough.) Continue with another sheet of phyllo, brushing with oil and creating an edge. After about 5 or 6 layers, you should have a nice-looking ruffled edge and a center area to fill with the tomatoes.

Start on the outside edge and arrange the tomatoes, fanning them together in a pattern, like the petals of a flower. Bake for 25 minutes, until the phyllo is brown on the edges.

Cut the tart into 6 squares and serve hot or at room temperature.

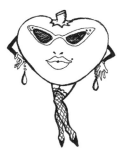

White Bean Garden Salad
LEVEL TWO

SERVES 8

This salad looks like a beautiful plant arrangement. Of course, you could bypass the garden look—simply toss all the ingredients together and serve. This Level Two recipe creates an imbalance because of the cheese and the beans.

4 cups cooked white beans (cannellini
  or small white navy beans)
¼ cup extra-virgin olive oil
3 garlic cloves, minced
Juice from 1 lemon
Salt and freshly ground black pepper

1 container radish sprouts
1 bunch fresh mint
2 medium tomatoes, diced
2 tablespoons drained capers
½ medium red onion, coarsely chopped
8 ounces feta cheese, crumbled

Place the beans in a serving dish and toss with the olive oil, garlic, lemon juice, salt, and pepper. Pretend you're planting a beautiful garden. Take a large handful of the radish sprouts and insert them into the beans as if they grew out of them. Then repeat the process with a handful of fresh mint, again placing it into the beans as if it sprouted from them.

Arrange the diced tomatoes on a separate area of the beans. Place the capers in a mound in another area. Place the red onions in another area. Finally, sprinkle the feta cheese around the other items. The end result should look like a beautiful potted garden. Make sure to include a taste of all the elements when you serve. Season with additional salt and pepper.

For Level One Carbos and Veggies Meal
Omit the olive oil and feta cheese. Add extra lemon juice if desired.

Whole Wheat Pasta with Pine Nuts

SERVES 4 TO 6

I discovered this quick and delicious meal on a night when I had nothing in the house to make for dinner. Combining these few ingredients made a great dish that Alan and I now eat frequently on Level Two. The combination of whole wheat pasta with oil and nuts creates a modest imbalance, but I find my system can handle it as long as I don't add any meat.

¼ cup olive oil
6 garlic cloves, minced
½ cup pine nuts
1 bunch flat-leaf parsley, chopped

Salt and freshly ground black pepper
1 pound cooked whole wheat pasta
    (linguine or spaghetti)

Heat the olive oil in a large skillet. Add the garlic and cook until lightly browned, about 3 minutes. Add the pine nuts, then the parsley, salt, and pepper. Continue stirring until the pine nuts start to brown.

In a large saucepan, cook the pasta until al dente; drain, reserving 3 tablespoons of the water. Add the pasta and 3 tablespoons water to the sauce and toss until heated through and completely coated.

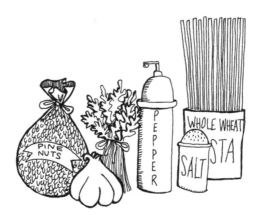

Whole Wheat Popovers

LEVEL TWO

MAKES 8 POPOVERS

These popovers are wonderful with a green salad for a light and delicious lunch. Popovers are muffin-size bread with a crisp crust and a puffy, moist inside. The mixture of Carbos (nonfat milk and whole wheat flour) and Proteins/Fats (butter and eggs) makes this a Level Two recipe.

1 cup nonfat milk
1 tablespoon melted butter
1 cup whole wheat pastry flour

¼ teaspoon salt
2 large eggs

Preheat the oven to 450°F. Butter a popover pan or a muffin tin.

In a large bowl, beat the milk, butter, flour, and salt together until smooth. Add the eggs, one at a time, being careful not to overbeat them. Fill the popover or muffin cups three-fourths full. Bake for 15 minutes. Without opening the oven door, turn the heat down to 350°F and bake an additional 20 minutes. Serve immediately.

Whole Wheat Pastry Crust

LEVEL TWO

❖

MAKES ONE 9-INCH SHELL

This crust combines Proteins/Fats and Carbos and it also has a little sugar. But it's certainly not as bad as a white flour pastry crust—if you're in the mood for a little indulgence, at least this is easier on your system. Frankly, I like the taste of this crust better than a standard crust. It's earthier and has more texture to offset the creamy fillings.

1 cup whole wheat pastry flour
2 tablespoons sugar
½ teaspoon salt
6 tablespoons butter, softened

1 egg yolk
½ teaspoon vanilla extract
1 tablespoon lemon juice

In a mixing bowl, combine the flour, sugar, and salt. Add the softened butter and work together with your fingertips or a pastry blender. Make a well in the center of the mixture (push the flour mixture to the sides of the bowl) and add the egg yolk, vanilla, and lemon juice. Mix the wet ingredients together with your fingertips and slowly incorporate the dry ingredients until the dough forms a ball and no longer adheres to your hands. Cover with waxed paper and refrigerate for at least 30 minutes.

Preheat the oven to 400° F. Butter and flour a 9-inch tart or pie pan.

Roll out the chilled dough on a floured board (see Note). Place the dough into the pie or tart pan and bake for 7 to 10 minutes, until golden brown.

Note Sometimes whole wheat doughs can be difficult to roll out. It you have a problem, simply press the dough with your fingertips into the pie or tart pan.

Double this recipe if you want a tip crust or lattice weave.

Berry Pie

LEVEL TWO

SERVES 6 TO 8

Every year for Alan's birthday, he asks our daughter-in-law, Caroline, to make her incredible berry pie. Once, when she set it out to cool after it came out of the oven, Alan and I inhaled the aroma and licked our lips. My son, Bruce, jokingly said, "Wouldn't it be great to eat the pie before dinner?" What a good idea! Before you knew it, the pie was completely gone. It's that wonderful.

2 tablespoons cornstarch
¼ cup orange juice
⅓ to ½ cup sugar, depending on sweetness
  of berries

6 cups fresh or frozen berries (any kind
  or combination; I like raspberries and
  blackberries)
Double recipe Whole Wheat Pastry Crust
  dough (opposite), in 2 pieces

Preheat the oven to 400°F.

Mix the cornstarch with the orange juice until smooth. Add the sugar and blend until well combined. Gently toss the berries with this mixture and let sit for about 15 minutes.

Grease a pie pan and line it with half the dough. Pierce the dough with a fork in several places. Bake for 7 to 10 minutes or until the crust is lightly browned. Remove the pie pan and turn up the oven to 450°F.

Place the berries in the bottom crust. Cover with a top crust, making slits to let out the steam (or make a lattice top, if you prefer). Bake for 10 minutes. Reduce the heat to 350°F and bake for 45 minutes, until juices are thickened and bubbly. Cool for a few hours before cutting and serving.

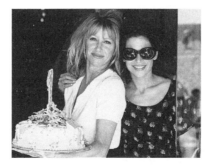

Me and my stepdaughter, Leslie, on her daughter Daisy's first birthday.

Lemon Curd Tart

LEVEL TWO

❖

SERVES 6 TO 8

A light and delicious tangy tart. To maintain my weight, I usually eat a Level One dinner and then enjoy this yummy tart for dessert. You can also make individual tartlets instead of one tart.

3 tablespoons butter, softened
¼ cup honey
2 large eggs, lightly beaten
¼ cup fresh lemon juice
Grated rind of 2 lemons

Whole Wheat Pastry Crust (page 194), cooled
Mint sprig or small edible flowers (pansies or nasturtium) for garnish

Blend the butter and the honey in a double boiler (or in a bowl or smaller saucepan placed over a saucepan of boiling water). When well combined, mix in the eggs, stirring constantly. Add the lemon juice and rind. Continue stirring until the custard thickens and coats the back of a wooden spoon.

Fill the crust with the lemon curd and garnish with a sprig of mint or flowers. Set aside until the curd is set. Tastes best when served at room temperature.

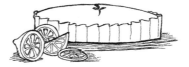

Fresh Berry Custard Tart

LEVEL TWO

SERVES 6

If you are trying to maintain your weight, you can eat a Level One dinner and then enjoy a piece of this delicious tart.

½ cup sugar
¼ cup cornstarch
4 egg yolks
2 cups whole milk
½ teaspoon vanilla extract

Whole Wheat Pastry Crust (page 194), cooled
2 cups mixed fresh berries, such as blackberries, raspberries, strawberries, or boysenberries

Combine ¼ cup of the sugar and all of the cornstarch in a mixing bowl and blend with a fork until smooth. Add the egg yolks and ½ cup of the milk, forming a paste. Put the remaining 1½ cups milk and ¼ cup sugar in a saucepan and bring to a boil. Add the hot milk mixture to the cold ingredients, whisking constantly. Pour back into the pan and stir over medium heat until smooth and thick. Remove from heat and add the vanilla. Chill for 2 hours.

Filled the cooled crust with the chilled custard. Arrange the berries in a pretty pattern on top, and serve.

Frozen Chocolate Mousse

LEVEL TWO

SERVES 6 TO 8

This is my version of the delicious Chocolate Mousse Mizou made on the eve of Stephen and Olivia's wedding. Everyone loves this dessert. It is always elegant and beautiful. Be sure to serve it on your best china or in crystal fruit compote bowls. Even martini glasses look great.

12 ounces semisweet chocolate, chopped
¾ cup boiling water
8 large eggs, separated
4 tablespoons almond–flavored liqueur
   (or 1½ teaspoons almond extract)
Artificial sweetener, if desired

GARNISH

1 pint heavy cream
1 teaspoon vanilla extract
Artificial sweetener, if desired
Shavings of semisweet chocolate

Place the chocolate in a blender or food processor and blend until reduced to a powder. Add the boiling water and blend until smooth. Then add the egg yolks and liqueur and blend until well combined. (If you prefer your mousse a little sweeter, add artificial sweetener at this point.)

In a separate bowl, beat the egg whites until they form stiff peaks. Using a large spatula, fold the chocolate mixture into the egg whites. Make large circular motions to blend thoroughly without deflating the egg whites.

Pour the mousse into a 2-quart freezer-proof bowl and freeze for at least 4 hours before serving. Take the mousse out of the freezer 1 hour before serving and keep it in the refrigerator. It should reach the consistency of soft ice cream.

Before serving, whip the cream with the vanilla until soft peaks form. (Add artificial sweetener, if desired.) Serve the frozen chocolate mousse with a dollop of whipped cream and a sprinkling of chocolate shavings.

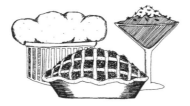

Chocolate Soufflé with Whipped Cream and Hot Chocolate Sauce

LEVEL TWO

SERVES 4 TO 6

Isn't this a difficult way to maintain your weight? I still find it hard to believe I can indulge myself like this. I love it! Use chocolate made from at least 60 percent cocoa.

SOUFFLÉ

4 ounces dark chocolate
3 egg yolks
5 tablespoons sugar
5 egg whites

HOT CHOCOLATE SAUCE

6 ounces dark chocolate, chopped
¾ cup heavy cream

WHIPPED CREAM

1 cup heavy cream
1 teaspoon vanilla extract
Artificial sweetener, if desired

Preheat the oven to 400°F. Butter a 1-quart soufflé dish.

For the soufflé: Melt the chocolate in a double boiler (or in a bowl or smaller saucepan placed over a bigger saucepan of boiling water). In a bowl, beat the egg yolks until they are pale yellow, then add the sugar. Continue to beat until well blended. Remove the chocolate from the heat and slowly add the egg mixture to the chocolate mixture. You don't want the eggs to cook.

In a separate bowl, beat the egg whites until they are stiff. Pour the chocolate mixture into the egg whites and fold gently with a spatula, using wide circular motions so that you keep as much air in the mixture as possible. Gently pour the mixture into the buttered soufflé dish and bake for 15 minutes.

For the chocolate sauce: Place the chopped chocolate in a bowl. Place the cream in a saucepan and bring to a boil. Add the hot cream to the chocolate and stir until all the lumps are gone.

For the whipped cream: Combine the cream and vanilla and whip either with an electric mixer or by hand with a whisk until soft peaks form. (Add a little artificial sweetener if you like.)

When the soufflé is done, serve immediately with a spoonful of hot chocolate sauce and a dollop of whipped cream.

Decadent Chocolate Cake

LEVEL TWO

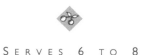

SERVES 6 TO 8

This rich and fudgy cake is made with whole wheat pastry flour and only a small amount of sugar. It's absolutely incredible and easier on the system than a standard chocolate cake with sugary butter-cream frosting. Use chocolate made from at least 60 percent cocoa.

CAKE

7½ ounces dark chocolate, chopped
11 tablespoons unsalted butter
4 large eggs, separated
⅓ cup sugar
⅓ cup whole wheat pastry flour

GANACHE

6 ounces dark chocolate, chopped
¾ cup heavy cream

Preheat the oven to 350°F. Butter and flour a 10-inch round cake pan.

For the cake: Melt the chocolate and butter in a double boiler (or in a bowl or smaller saucepan placed over a saucepan of boiling water). Set aside to cool.

Beat the egg yolks until light and fluffy. Slowly add the sugar and continue beating until mixture is pale yellow. Fold in the melted chocolate. Sift the flour over the chocolate mixture until it just disappears.

In a separate bowl, whisk the egg whites until soft peaks form. Fold egg whites into the chocolate mixture in 2 parts. Pour the batter into the prepared pan and tap on the counter to remove air bubbles. Bake for 20 to 25 minutes, until a toothpick comes out clean (see Note).

For the ganache: Place the chopped chocolate in a mixing bowl. Place the cream in a saucepan and bring to a boil. Add the hot cream to the chocolate and stir until all lumps are gone. Let the ganache stand until it reaches room temperature, then pour it over the cooled cake and spread with a spatula.

Note For a thicker cake, double the recipe and bake for 35 minutes.

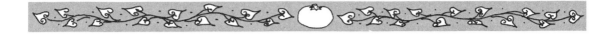

Afterword

As you have learned from these recipes, Somersizing allows you to eat and stay slim in a way you've never before dreamed possible. People are always asking me how I've been able to maintain my desired weight and yet eat foods that are normally forbidden on traditional "diets." Somersizing is a healthy new way to eat, a way of life to embrace forever. I am grateful to have created this program for myself and I am so pleased to share it with you.

Now that you understand how it works, I am sure you will want to share it with your friends. With your new figure comes a renewed sense of self-confidence. You set out to achieve a goal and you have. Enjoy the compliments; you worked hard for them and you should be proud of yourself. Enjoy your meals, enjoy your new body, and enjoy your new lifestyle.

Somersizing has been a truly liberating experience for me and I hope that in sharing it with you, your life has been enhanced in some way—either through losing a few pounds or in learning some new tricks in the kitchen. Congratulations. It's been a pleasure Somersizing with you!

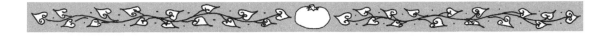

Index

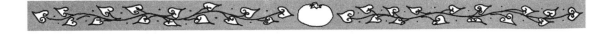

About the Author

Suzanne Somers, a symbol of fitness and health, is the author of the best-selling book *Keeping Secrets*. She lectures nationally on the effects of addiction on families. The star of the long-running sitcom *Step by Step* and the former star of *Three's Company,* she is a Las Vegas entertainer and was named Entertainer of the Year in 1987, along with Frank Sinatra. She is also the spokesperson for and owner of the wildly successful ThighMaster fitness products.

CONVERSION CHART
EQUIVALENT IMPERIAL AND METRIC MEASUREMENTS

American cooks use standard containers, the 8-ounce cup and a tablespoon that takes exactly 16 level fillings to fill that cup level. Measuring by cup makes it very difficult to give weight equivalents, as a cup of densely packed butter will weigh considerably more than a cup of flour. The easiest way therefore to deal with cup measurements in recipes is to take the amount by volume rather than by weight. Thus the equation reads:

1 cup = 240 ml = 8 fl. oz.   1/2 cup = 120 ml = 4 fl. oz.

It is possible to buy a set of American cup measures in major stores around the world.

In the States, butter is often measured in sticks. One stick is the equivalent of 8 tablespoons. One tablespoon of butter is therefore the equivalent to ½ ounce/15 grams.

SOLID MEASURES

U.S. and Imperial Measures		Metric Measures	
Ounces	Pounds	Grams	Kilos
1		28	
2		56	
3½		100	
4	¼	112	
5		140	
6		168	
8	½	225	
9		250	¼
12	¾	340	
16	1	450	
18		500	½
20	1¼	560	
24	1½	675	
27		750	¾
28	1¾	780	
32	2	900	
36	2¼	1000	1
40	2½	1100	
48	3	1350	
54		1500	1½
64	4	1800	
72	4½	2000	2
80	5	2250	2¼
90		2500	2½
100	6	2800	2¾

LIQUID MEASURES

Fluid Ounces	U.S.	Imperial	Milliliters
	1 teaspoon	1 teaspoon	5
¼	2 teaspoons	1 dessertspoon	10
½	1 tablespoon	1 tablespoon	14
1	2 tablespoons	2 tablespoons	28
2	¼ cup	4 tablespoons	56
4	½ cup		110
5		¼ pint or 1 gill	140
6	¾ cup		170
8	1 cup		225
9			250
10	1¼ cups	½ pint	280
12	1½ cups		340
15		¾ pint	420
16	2 cups		450
18	2¼ cups		500
20	2½ cups	1 pint	560
24	3 cups		675
25		1¼ pints	700
27	3½ cups		750
30	3¾ cups	1½ pints	840
32	4 cups or 1 quart		900
35		1¾ pints	980
36	4½ cups		1000
40	5 cups	2 pints or 1 quart	1120
48	6 cups		1350
50		2½ pints	1400
60	7½ cups	3 pints	1680
64	8 cups or 2 quarts		1800
72	9 cups		2000

OVEN TEMPERATURE EQUIVALENTS

Fahrenheit	Celsius	Gas Mark	Description
225	110	¼	Cool
250	130	½	
275	140	1	Very Slow
300	150	2	
325	170	3	Slow
350	180	4	Moderate
375	190	5	
400	200	6	Moderately Hot
425	220	7	Fairly Hot
450	230	8	Hot
475	240	9	Very Hot
500	250	10	Extremely Hot

EQUIVALENTS FOR INGREDIENTS

all-purpose flour—plain flour
arugula—rocket
confectioners' sugar—icing sugar
cornstarch—cornflour
eggplant—aubergine
granulated sugar—castor sugar
half and half—12% fat milk
lima beans—broad beans
scallion—spring onion
shortening—white fat
squash—courgettes or marrow
unbleached flour—strong, white flour
vanilla bean—vanilla pod
zest—rind
zucchini—courgettes

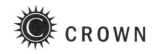